Periodontal Care for Older Adults

Hosted by

Canadian Academy of Periodontology
and
Department of Periodontics
University of Toronto

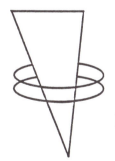

May 10th & 11th 1991

Richard P. Ellen, Editor

This Symposium was supported by a generous educational grant from **Colgate-Palmolive Canada** and a grant from the **Ontario Ministry of Health.**

Periodontal Care for Older Adults

First published in 1992 by
Canadian Scholars' Press Inc.
339 Bloor Street West, Suite 220
Toronto, M5S 1W7
Canada

Canadian Cataloguing in Publication Data

Main entry under title:

Periodontal Care for Older Adults

ISBN 0-921627-73-4

1. Periodontal disease - Congresses. 2. Aged - Dental care-Congresses. 3. I. Ellen, Richard P., 1946-.

RK361.A2P47 1992   618.97'7632   C91-094124-6

Cover design by Kaerynne Pohlak
Book design by The Dancing Puffin Co.

...to my parents, Selda and Harry Ellen, and their generation of adults who are chronologically older than I....

Contributors

Sharon M. Aitken, Research Associate, Department of Periodontics, Faculty of Dentistry, University of Toronto.

Pierre Baehni, Professor of Preventive Dentistry, Faculty of Medicine, University of Geneva.

David W. Banting, Professor and Associate Dean (Academic), University of Western Ontario, Chief of Staff, Parkwood Hospital, London, Ontario,

Bruce J. Baum, Director of the Clinical Investigation Branch of the National Institute of Dental Research, U.S.A.

James D. Beck, Professor and Chairperson, Department of Dental Ecology, University of North Carolina.

Peter Birek, Associate Professor, Department of Periodontics, University of Toronto.

Laura J. Dempster, Tutor, Faculty of Dentistry, University of Toronto, Department of Preventive Dentistry.

Richard P. Ellen, Professor of Dentistry and Microbiology, Head of the Department of Periodontics, Faculty of Dentistry, University of Toronto.

Ronald L. Ettinger, Professor, Department of Prosthodontics, Dows Institute for Dental Research, University of Iowa.

Roy S. Feldman, Chief, Dental Service, Philadelphia V.A. Medical Center, Adjunct Associate Professor of Periodontology, School of Dental Medicine, University of Pennsylvania.

Margery G.E. Forgay, Acting Director, School of Dental Hygiene, University of Manitoba.

Sidney Golden, Assistant Professor, Department of Periodontics, Faculty of Dentistry, University of Toronto.

Tim Gould, Associate Professor, Division of Periodontics, Director, Graduate/Postgraduate Program in Periodontics, University of British Columbia.

Helen A. Grad, Clinical Pharmacologist, Faculty of Dentistry, University of Toronto.

Daniel A. Haas, Assistant Professor, Department of Anaesthesia, Faculty of Dentistry, University of Toronto, Department of Pharmacology, Faculty of Medicine.

Marc W. Heft, Director of the Claude Denson Pepper Center for Research on Oral Health in Aging, Associate Professor, Department of Oral and Maxillofacial Surgery, College of Dentistry, University of Florida.

Patricia M. Johnson, Professor of the Dental Health Programs, Seneca College of Applied Arts and Technology, Toronto.

Daniel Kandelman, Professor and Chairman, Division of Preventive and Community Dentistry, Faculty of Dentistry, University of Montreal.

H. Asuman Kiyak, Professor, Department of Oral and Maxillofacial Surgery, Adjunct Professor, Department of Psychology, University of Washington.

David M. Kogon, Health Care Consultant, William M. Mercer Ltd., Canada.

James L. Leake, Professor and Head, Department of Community Dentistry, Faculty of Dentistry, University of Toronto, Dental Director, East York Health Unit.

Hardy Limeback, Associate Professor, Department of Preventive Dentistry, Faculty of Dentistry, University of Toronto, Chief of Dental Services, Metropolitan Toronto Homes for the Aged.

David Locker, Professor, Department of Community Dentistry, Faculty of Dentistry, University of Toronto.

Harald Löe, Director, National Institute of Dental Research, National Institute of Health, U.S.A.

Walter J. Loesche, Professor of Dentistry, Professor of Microbiology, School of Medicine, University of Michigan.

Mai Pohlak, Coordinator of Continuing Dental Education, Senior Tutor, Department of Preventive Dentistry, Faculty of Dentistry, University of Toronto.

Nils Ravald, Chief, Specialty Clinic in Periodontics, Linköping, Sweden, Research Scientist, Department of Cariology, University of Göteborg, Sweden.

Paul B. Robertson, Dean, Professor of Clinical Dentistry Sciences, Faculty of Dentistry, University of British Columbia.

Adrianne M. Schmitt, Assistant Professor, Department of Prosthodontics, Faculty of Dentistry, University of Toronto.

Jonathan Ship, Senior Investigator, Clinical Coordinator Oral Medicine Training Program, NIDR, U.S.A.

Michael J. Sigal, Associate Professor, Department of Pediatric Dentistry, Faculty of Dentistry, University of Toronto, Chief of Dentistry, Queen Elizabeth Hospital.

David L. Sumney, Clinical Associate Professor, School of Dental Medicine, University of Pittsburgh, Clinical Assistant Professor of Medicine, Medical College of Pennsylvania, Senior Attending, Department of Medicine, Allegheny General Hospital.

Table of Contents

Part 2: Opinion

Preface

Aging is much more than the accumulation of years. It is the accumulation of events. It is the accumulation of joys and the accumulation of tragedies. It is the accumulation of creativity and the accumulation of habits. It is the accumulation of submissiveness and the accumulation of stubbornness. Marketing experts, who sell dreams, will say that it is the accumulation of wealth, but observers of reality know it to be the accumulation of poverty for far too many. Aging is also the accumulation of wrinkles, medications, and minor ailments. It can be at once the hardening of the arteries and the hardening of perceptions...the accumulation of scars. Aging: irreversible accumulations, both physical and behavioral. The key features of periodontitis, loss of connective tissue attachment and resorption of supporting alveolar bone, are essentially irreversible if allowed to progress naturally. Therefore, the signs and severity of periodontal disease also accumulate with advancing age, along with the biological, behavioral, and perceptual factors which have caused it.

Periodontal Care for Older Adults is based on the proceedings of a symposium of the same title which was held at the University of Toronto on May 10 and 11, 1991. It was a unique event, co-hosted by The Canadian Academy of Periodontology and The Department of Periodontics of the University of Toronto, Faculty of Dentistry. Over 200 health professionals, who care for and about the dental needs of older adults, met and debated a series of key issues which, in essence, can be expressed by the very clever title chosen by one of the principal speaker/authors: "Periodontal Services for Older Adults; What They Need and What They Get."

Like the symposium, the book is divided into two parts. The charge of the first day of the symposium was *information*. The first part of the book consists of manuscripts detailing the lecture-style presentations of principal speaker/authors who are authorities with minds-on/hands-on experience in the field. The charge of the second day was *opinion*; smaller group workshops offered a forum in which panels of provocative discussants provoked the participants to debate assigned topics and formulate strong suggestions for future directions. The second part of the book consists of manuscripts co-authored by the panelists, including summaries of the major points of discussion as presented by the panel leader to the plenary session.

The success of both symposium and book depend on the expertise, dedication, and style of the speakers, panelists, and participants. I recognise and salute them. I would also like to express my appreciation to the eight postgraduate residents in my department, who played an outstanding role in coordinating the activities of the discussion groups: C. Allison, G. Galli, E. Nemeth, G. Romanelli, F. Sun, Y.-T. A. Teng, J.-F. Tessier and M.C. Traversy. I am grateful to Mai Pohlak and Jennifer White of the Faculty of Dentistry's Continuing Education Department for careful attention to details in the organization of the symposium. Ending at the beginning, I wish to thank Professor J.R.S. Prichard, President of the University of Toronto, and Dr. M. Budd, representing the officers of the Canadian Academy of Periodontology, for joining me in welcoming the participants to the symposium. They and I, along with the speakers and panelists, now take pleasure in welcoming you, the readers of our book.

RPE, 1991

Part 1: Information

Chapters 1–9 are single-authored chapters based on lecture-style presentations on the first day of the symposium. The authors were instructed both to review the assigned field and to color the presentation with individual analysis and provocation. The themes developed in these chapters were to carry through to the workshop group discussions, which are summarized in chapters 10–17.

Chapter 1
Keynote: Issues in Geriatric Dentistry

Harald Löe

Aging is news these days. We are continually astonished by the latest figures on how many "old" and "old-old" "and oldest old" there are; how many more there will be by the year so-and-so. Many view these demographic imperatives with alarm: As the elderly increase, so does the prevalence of Alzheimer's disease, other dementia, heart disease, strokes, cancers, and accidents—mostly from falls, in the case of older people. All that pain and suffering translates to more nursing homes, more high-tech medicine, more intensive care units, and all the attendant direct and indirect costs that drive nations' health budgets to astronomical heights.

From another perspective, however, the fact that there are more people surviving clearly is cause for rejoicing. Not all old people are candidates for organ transplants or total hip replacements—or dentures for that matter, and not all are "losing it" mentally. Most older Americans live independently; many are in retirement homes in circumstances that are quite adequate. In other words, for many, the quality of life is excellent.

For *many*, but clearly not for all. The real concerns and the major questions for biological research today are: why can't all of us live longer and healthier lives and if not (which is clearly the case) what can be done about it? Today, the average lifespan in North America is approximately 75 years—an enormous increase in the course of a century—for which we credit improved socio-economic circumstances, better hygiene, better nutrition, and the control of most infectious diseases. These factors alone have created what some are calling a new age in history: the AGE age.

But 75 is no endpoint in the lifespan. There are already 3 million U.S. citizens over the age of 85, and the estimate is that there may be as many as 50 million by the middle of the 21st century. The question is: How much more life can we expect? Suppose we could wipe out chronic diseases; would people die of "old age?"

There are some well-known basic changes that occur in the course of "normal" aging that increase the risk of dying. I am thinking of declines in immune function, declines in the ability of cells to repair errors in DNA; and there are intracellular accumulations of toxic products that can lead to cellular malfunction or destruction. Over the years each of these phenomena has given rise to one or another theory of aging; however, as yet there is no consensus.

Others have postulated that the maximum lifespan of animals is programmed into the species according to certain rules. One rule was simply that big animals live longer than small ones; another was that animals with lower rates of metabolism outlive those with more rapid rates: the elephant versus the mouse. Georges Buffon, the 18th century French naturalist, extended these observations into a rule of thumb, that animals tend to live six times the period it takes for them to mature. For example, since it takes some 20 years for human beings to reach skeletal maturity—including the development of wisdom teeth—that would mean a maximum human lifespan of 120 years.

Modern refinements of the Buffon approach take into consideration the rate of development, the length of the reproductive period, maximum caloric consumption, and the size of the brain. Such calculations would yield a lifespan of 3 years for the house mouse, 70 for elephants, 100 for whales, and 110 for man—not at all unreasonable estimates.

Still another programming rule that has been applied to measuring the maximum lifespan looks at the rate of decline in function of vital organs over time. In the absence of disease, the decline is very gradual, on the order of 1 percent per year after the age of 30. Assuming 100 percent efficiency at age 30, and given the redundancy built into human organ systems, people would only begin to feel losses of function at age 100 or so.

The concept of a programmed maximum lifespan or, conversely, a programmed time of dying received a boost from the studies of Leonard Hayflick in the 1970s. Hayflick took human fibroblasts and counted the number of cell divisions that occurred in culture. As the cells approached 50 doublings they became senescent, stopped dividing, and died. Cells from older donors underwent fewer divisions. The cells seemed to follow an agenda of programmed cell death. While Hayflick readily admits that what happens in cell culture may not apply *in vivo,* calculations of the number of doublings multiplied by the cell life of each cell yield a figure close to 120 years as the maximum human lifespan. Thus, in the absence of disease, several lines of reasoning converge on a figure between 110 and 120 as the maximum human lifespan.

The concept of programmed cell death has gained increasing currency in recent years. Embryonic development is characterized by the proliferation of more cells than can possibly survive in the course of morphogenesis and organogenesis. Thus, developmental biologists speak of cells that are "programmed to die."

This characteristic also applies to immune cells. Studies of monocytes in circulation indicate that most senesce and die, and are removed by phagocytosis in the liver or spleen. However, this is a genetically programmed cell death that is different from the cellular swelling seen during necrosis of cells. The immune cells are said to commit suicide in an act called *apoptosis,* in which they shrink, their DNA becomes fragmented, and they become permeable to dyes.

Interestingly, these immune cell suicides can be prevented by the addition of a number of cytokines. Scientists at the National Institute of Dental Research (NIDR) have been exploring this phenomenon in the course of research on the basic features of inflammation, both in relation to periodontal disease and arthritic joints. As is well known, in a chronic inflammatory lesion immune cells remain alive at the site for a long time. Actually this fact is what gives name to and characterizes this pathological lesion: *chronic* inflammation. The working hypothesis is that the monocytes are prevented from suicide by immuno-stimulating factors like interleukin 1, gamma interferon, and possibly other cytokines. The logical next step is then to look for agents to block the production or action of these immune system factors which would prevent or reduce inflammation.

So, from a consideration of aging and programmed cell death we might arrive at a potential therapy for periodontal disease—one based on manipulating the body's own immune system. This, of course, is typical of the way that science works. It is why it is so important for all of us—and especially NIDR—to keep alive the idle curiosity that is the basis of scientific inquiry and to continue to support basic research into fundamental and generalisable mechanisms.

However, in spite of all we hear about longer lives, new revelations in science and the marvels of high-tech medicine, many people, even scientists working in the field, believe that aging is a dismal affair, a state of failing health and well-being. Or, as expressed in Shakespeare's memorable lines, "*sans* teeth, *sans* eyes, *sans* taste, *sans* everything." Underlying this pessimistic portrait of age, it seems to me, is a fundamental confusion between aging as such and aging in the context of general health conditions in the presence of systemic disease and disease treatments.

Applying some of the basic mechanisms of aging to the oral tissues that make up the mouth, teeth, and the jaws: the epithelia and connective tissues of the oral mucosa, the tongue, palate, gingiva and the periodontal ligament; all the mineralized tissues—enamel, dentin, cementum, and bone; and the neurological tissues providing for the sensory and motor functions of the oral structures, as well as the vasculature and the complex of tissues governing the production and secretion of saliva of various kinds—considering the incredible complexity of the oral-maxillo-facial organ and realizing that major basic data are still unavailable—I must conclude *that these structures and their function, individually or in concert, are surprisingly little influenced by aging per se.*

Sure, like skin, oral mucosa becomes less elastic because of changes in the collagen and other connective tissue matrix components. Yes, there are fewer cells and relatively more intercellular substance, and the interface between the epithelium and the connective tissue loses its undulation and the basement membrane flattens out—both in the oral mucosa and in the gingiva, but there are no indications that in general these changes have led to significant functional consequences. Cell turnover or replacement of epithelial cells is not significantly changed; keratinization, if changed, is probably increased and the reparative capacity of connective tissue during aging seems to be unaltered. Also, initiation of periodontal disease shows no significant difference to that in younger animals and humans.

Certainly, there are physiological changes in the tissues of the oral complex as a function of endocrinological fluctuations in women, also as they reach menopause and after. Osteoporosis occurs in the jaw bones as it does in the rest of the skeleton, but osteoporosis is a qualitative change impacting on the density of bone and does not influence the length of individual bones or the height of the alveolar bone.

Although gingival recession, loss of periodontal attachment, and reduction in alveolar bone are closely associated with age, there are no data suggesting that either has anything to do with aging. Passive eruption was once a concept that attempted to describe a physiological age change in the periodontium during which occlusal movement of the tooth and compensatory cementum formation occurred in response to occlusal attrition or loss of occluding antagonist. Since the theory further implied that during the occlusal movement of the tooth, no corresponding bone formation at the alveolar ridge took place, the net effect was a continuous reduction in periodontal attachment, including gingival recession, lengthening of the clinical crown, and increasing exposure of the roots of the teeth. The ultimate consequence of this concept was that the teeth, with age, would literally grow out of their sockets.

The whole idea sounds pretty unreasonable in this day and age, but at one time this was an important aspect of periodontal physiology. It is no longer, as we and others have shown, that as teeth move occlusally, they bring the alveolar bone with them. The only reason for bringing it up is that in the evolution of periodontal science, passive eruption represented a set of physiological changes that once were considered to be genuine age changes. With passive eruption rejected as a physiological and continuous process caused by aging *per se*, there is nothing in the realm of periodontal biology or physiology that I know of that would jeopardize the longevity of the supporting tissues of teeth. Also, I have seen no data that would support the notion that loss of teeth and edentulism has anything to do with the biological mechanism of aging. Tooth decay and its causes are unrelated to the aging process—although root surface caries occurs more frequently in older individuals. Salivary gland functions and saliva show no major changes during aging. Mastication and muscle function in older patients with teeth are relatively unaffected, taste sensations are not measurably reduced in old age and oral motor functions are relatively well preserved. So, what are we doing here in Toronto?

In 1986-87 NIDR conducted a national survey of the oral health situation of adult working Americans and senior citizens. Altogether, the sample counted approximately 25,000 individuals, 5000 of whom were persons 65 years of age and older. The survey told us that the young-to-middle aged cohorts are doing reasonably well. Adults reach maturity today with fewer cavities, although they continue to experience caries attacks through the third and fourth decades. Their periodontal situation is also improved as compared with age-mates some 10-15 years ago. Only 4 percent of the working population in the U.S. between 18 and 65 years old are edentulous or have lost all their teeth.

In contrast, the prevalence of toothlessness in the older age groups is 10 times higher: almost 50% of Americans 65 and older are missing all their teeth. Those who still have teeth continue to experience coronal caries at about the same rate as younger adults and have a prevalence of root caries that is three times greater than the working population.

Also, today's seniors have the most severe and extensive signs of periodontal disease of any age group examined. So, the oral health problems of the elderly are targets for concern. Furthermore, the senior citizens examined constitute relatively healthy people, healthy enough to attend senior citizens' centres where the dental examinations were held. We have very little data on the oral health status of the elderly who are homebound, institutionalized, handicapped, or who lack self care or access to services, but I would expect it is even worse. In other words, we have great numbers of old people whose oral health is terrible!

No one has a complete account of all the reasons for this miserable state of affairs, and surely the explanations are many and varied. Not only do we have to contend with the impact of various systemic diseases on oral health over a lifetime, or assorted systemic disease treatments which influence oral homeostasis; there are mental and physical handicaps to reckon with, and an array of socioeconomic variables, lifestyle and other factors that increase the risk for oral health problems.

However, it seems to me that one of the main reasons for the state of oral health in the current cohort of Americans is the fact that they grew up between the two world wars and amidst economic depression, with very little possibility to benefit from preventive approaches to dental care, even if they had the means and the inclination—because there was no preventive dentistry.

Tooth loss, although the ultimate measure of how well we in science and practice are succeeding in controlling oral diseases, is not only a function of disease. Tooth mortality also reflects socioeconomic conditions, individual and cultural circumstances, as well as already mentioned, the knowledge base underlying past standards of care. What all this means is that the magnitude of oral health and oral care problems of older adults in America, Canada and other developed countries is probably greater today than it will be in the future. However, we cannot be certain that a mere cohort effect is going to take care of the elderly of a distant future. Even if it will, we need solutions for tomorrow's elderly.

That, in a nutshell, is exactly what we are aiming to do in the *NIDR Research and Action Program for Improving the Oral health of Older Americans and Other Adults at High Risk*. As many of you would know, we started this activity several years ago at the time we had the first results of the adult survey. We said then that the time was right for an expansion of the research agenda from a sole concern for primary caries prevention in schoolchildren to a concern for the whole spectrum of oral health problems of children, adults, and old people.

That concern carries a mandate to study the oral aspects of normal development, maturity, and aging, as well as research on the various oral conditions and how they affect and are affected by systemic disease and disease treatments. Most importantly, we need to get on with the job of finding out who is at risk and why. That means basic molecular biology and more analytical epidemiology studies, risk factor analysis, and behavioral and social science research. It means looking at disadvantaged groups, members of minorities, and the sick and frail. It includes a review of what is taught and learned in dental school, and it has to do with clinical decisions and attitudes in dental practice.

We have already begun these studies; indeed, we are moving ahead on all aspects of the program. The U.S. Congress is extremely interested, the U.S. Public Health Service has pledged its support, and the private sector has gotten involved. A private foundation has established a Steering Committee to guide a major national disease prevention/oral health promotion campaign.

Over the last 150 years dentistry in industrialized societies has evolved in three phases: First, there was a preoccupation with relieving pain and pulling teeth. Second, we developed technologies that enabled us to save teeth by filling cavities. Third is the phase that Western dentistry is entering in full force: prevention. Only now have we reached this phase, and only because we are able to take advantage of what research has taught us about the causes of oral diseases. These advances allow us to get on with the job of prevention in all its complexity.

Furthermore, the growth and expansion of dental science means that prevention research and activities are going beyond the traditional dental disorders to include all the disorders and diseases affecting the face, the mouth, and the jaws, as well as all the systemic diseases, systemic disease treatments, and conditions that have consequences for oral care. However, the realization of why they are important and the communication of that information to the public and the patient ultimately rests on the dental professionals. If we are to capitalize on the broadening of the research agenda we must ensure that the schools broaden the curricula to educate tomorrow's dentists.

We need more internal medicine, more genetics and molecular biology, more clinical pharmacology, and more emphasis on normal aging and geriatrics. To go along with the needs of older patients as well as those with general disease or handicaps, we need an increased emphasis on behavioral science, communication skills, and clinical decision-making. At the same time, we need to revitalize traditional elements in the curriculum, such as more sophisticated restorative dentistry. We need to emphasize the newer tooth-conserving materials and methods. All this translates to a need to ensure that new technologies for prevention, diagnosis, and early intervention are integrated into the curriculum.

These are exciting developments in the history of dentistry, indeed of all the health professions. Progress in understanding the transition from health to disease and from disease to health has gained enormously as we have passed from the level of the organism, the tissue, the cell and now the molecule. But the reverse journey is equally important. Once we have a handle on the cell and molecular derangements in disease processes, we must go up the scale to engage the whole organism in the healing process. Beyond the whole organism there is society itself, and the community of societies that constitutes the world today—a world where people can live longer and richer lives, and with their natural teeth over the natural lifetime.

Chapter 2
Epidemiology of Periodontal Diseases in Older Adults

James D. Beck

I. Introduction

Being asked to do a review of the epidemiology of periodontal diseases is akin to being commissioned to write a book about an unsolved mystery. Fortunately, it is to be a short story, because I was given a very explicit focus for this endeavour, to discuss epidemiologic evidence of risk factors for periodontal diseases in older adults. The first question to be answered in gathering material for this assignment is to see if we can uncover the facts upon which this short story is to be based. In order to do this properly, I first need to describe the setting by presenting some issues pertaining to the identification of risk factors; issues involved in comparing data from different epidemiologic studies; and issues pertaining to aging. In light of the issues discussed, a summary of findings from studies reported in the literature during the last five years on the prevalence of periodontal diseases and potential risk indicators will be presented. These findings will be followed by current data on the incidence of periodontal attachment loss and possible risk factors.

Issues in Risk Assessment

The development of risk models has two distinct phases: risk factor identification and model development. Statistical considerations in developing risk models have been reviewed by Koch and Beck[1] and additional issues involving risk factor identification have been reviewed by Beck.[2] At the outset, researchers must decide which types of risk models they wish to develop.

For most medical conditions and diseases an individual either contracts it or does not, thereby making the selection of the dichotomous outcome model the appropriate choice. However, periodontitis exhibits a pattern of multiple attacks in which an individual can contract the condition multiple times; reoccurring at the same site or occurring in multiple different sites. This problem of multiple disease attack seen in periodontitis influences definitions of what level of disease intensity constitutes "high risk". Dental measurements usually are made on sites or surfaces, but risk is assigned to the individual. This difference between the unit of analysis and the unit of measurement results in researchers summing up the number of sites or surfaces attacked in each individual, resulting in a distribution of people based on the total number of sites or surfaces that have experienced periodontitis.

A decision must be made among several options on how to define high risk. Does one follow (1) the medical model of "presence or absence" of the disease; (2) define high risk as the upper 5, 10, 15, etc. percent of the distribution of attack across sites and surfaces; (3) determine a clinically significant cut-point; or (4) use some combination of these definitions. Since the goal of risk assessment is to predict new disease, the choice of a definition will be influenced by the incidence of the disease, the perceived seriousness of the disease, and what is to be predicted. Criterion-based definitions (presence or absence, clinically significant) are more comparable across studies than population-based definitions that depend on the distribution of disease in the study population. For the same disease or condition, a "presence or absence" definition of high risk may result in a different risk model than a "gradient" definition. People who are susceptible to a generalized disease attack in the mouth may have different risk factors than those who only experience disease at a single site, or the factors may interact differently.

Prediction models usually contain two types of predictors; indicators and risk factors[2]. Indicators are variables that are not believed to be etiologic for the disease of interest. Prevalence studies will only allow the testing of associations. Causal interpretations from these associations are tenuous and must follow the guidelines set forth by Lilienfeld[3]. Therefore, associations derived from prevalence studies should not be thought of as risk factors, but as potential risk factors or risk indicators. Although many methodologists indicate that something cannot truly be called a risk factor until it has been found to influence disease in a clinical or community trial, factors found to be associated with the incidence of disease, with support from clinical and laboratory studies, often are considered to be risk factors. This discussion will take the latter approach in discussing risk factors. Furthermore, our knowledge about what is a causal factor is constantly changing and it is possible that some indicator variables will eventually be classified as causal (etiologic) and vice versa.

Some indicators, such as baseline number of teeth, can be powerful predictors of who will experience attachment loss without being direct causes of the condition. On the other hand, the term "risk factor" implies causality. Models are restricted to risk factors (causal factors) when the objective is to identify the relationships and relative strengths of multiple causes of a disease in order to develop the most effective prevention or treatment intervention. These are called etiologic models. However, when the objective is to maximize the ability of the model to identify high risk and low risk individuals (maximize sensitivity and specificity), models allowing both indicators and risk factors are usually employed. These are called prediction models. While prediction models may perform better than etiologic models, they may contain variables that will not influence the incidence of disease if changed. In addition, the presence of powerful indicators in a model may mask the effects of related etiologic factors. For example, the presence of periodontal pockets in a model may be highly correlated with the presence of microorganisms in the model.

Issues in Comparing Epidemiologic Studies of Periodontal Diseases

Normally, when we want to know about the epidemiology of a disease or condition, we want to know the prevalence of the disease (how much is out there), the incidence of the disease (how much new disease can we expect in a given time period), and the characteristics of people most at risk for the disease. Usually, no one study can provide all this information; so we attempt to derive estimates from a number of studies. In order to properly estimate disease prevalence and incidence from a number of studies, those studies should be roughly comparable, especially in the manner in which they measure the disease. Thus, it is useful to review some of the measures used in various studies to get a feel for how comparable the studies are.

Clinical Trials and Population-Based Studies

Studies involving some type of sampling frame to represent a larger population can provide unbiased estimates of prevalence and incidence, with proper weighting for the sampling design and unbiased responses. In contrast, clinical trials usually are select populations designed to maximize the likelihood of finding differences between two therapies and thus may not be representative of a general population of interest. This review concentrates on those studies that are population based, except in those instances where baseline data on clinical studies were drawn from populations rather than patients.

Indices of Periodontal Disease Used

Epidemiologic indices of periodontal diseases have evolved along with our understanding of the nature of the disease. We have moved from indices like the Periodontal Index,[4] which encompasses both gingivitis and periodontitis, to disaggregated measures such as pocket depth, gingival recession, and attachment loss. The problem presented is that any review of changing disease patterns over time must confront the comparison of disease measured by the PI, with disease measured in terms of pocket depth or attachment loss. The matter is further complicated by the manner in which the different indices are employed in studies. In some studies, pocket depth or attachment loss is measured only on selected teeth or on randomly selected quadrants of the mouth, rather than on all teeth. At the tooth level, some studies measure and record at one or two sites, while other studies measure at six sites per tooth. The prime concern with these types of comparisons is whether or not the epidemiologic data are conservative measures of disease. In general, it appears that partial recording of mouths or sites does not underestimate average pocket depths or average loss of attachment, but it does underestimate the prevalence (percent of people) of disease, especially the less frequently occurring serious disease.

Definition of a "Case"

In epidemiology, the definition of what is and what is not a "case" of a disease is critical; it can lead to threats to internal validity of the study, and it may make comparison of prevalence rates across studies a tenuous proposition. As an example, Bergstrom and Eliasson[5] show that different case definitions for probing pocket depth can have dramatic effects on the estimated prevalence (or incidence) of disease.

Types of Information to be Presented

This review of the epidemiology of periodontal diseases will concentrate on studies of a population or studies using a sampling frame to estimate disease in a population. Pretreatment baseline data or data from nontreated control groups in clinical trials will be used only if they represent populations and not groups of patients. Studies using comparable definitions of a "case" will be used or differences will be noted.

As knowledge about the intraoral distribution of disease has changed as a result of the use of more objective field measures, as described above, the small number of diseased sites per person, even in populations with a high prevalence, has led to concern that the use of mean scores per subject may obscure changes that occur at these few sites. Thus, this review will concentrate on measures of prevalence and incidence that do not employ mean scores and will concentrate on studies that do not assume independence of sites when identifying risk indicators or risk factors.

Finally, this review will only report on longitudinal studies that measure disease in terms of amount of attachment loss. This is done for several reasons. We are interested in risk factors for periodontitis, which implies the use of longitudinal study designs. Since attachment loss makes use of a fixed reference point, it is thought to be the better clinical measure of disease progression.[6,7] Attachment loss will be emphasized as a measure of the prevalence of disease, but there are a limited number of prevalence studies that report attachment loss. Consequently, pocket depth also will be used as a measure of disease prevalence. Where partial mouth recording and number of sites examined appear to affect prevalence estimates, it will be noted. Since the Community Periodontal Index of Treatment Needs (CPITN)[8] does record pocket depth, but was designed as an index of treatment needs rather than as a measure of disease, only a few studies using this measure are included to provide comparisons of prevalence rates reported.

Issues in Studying Aging

We currently lack precise knowledge of what constitutes normal aging. Much of our information comes from cross-sectional studies, which compare findings from a group of younger people with those from a group of older people. Such data may reflect differences other than the effects of age. The older people represent a cohort of survivors. Many changes associated with aging result from gradual loss. These losses may begin early in childhood. Currently, we think in terms of the one percent rule; most organ systems seem to lose function at roughly one percent a year beginning at age 30. However, newer data show that in some organ systems, such as the kidney, a subgroup of people appear to experience gradually declining function over time, whereas others' function remains constant. If these findings are substantiated, the earlier theory of gradual loss must be reassessed as reflecting disease rather than aging. Thus, the ideas of what constitutes normal aging is constantly being reassessed. We must keep the concept of separating normal aging from periodontal disease in mind as we deal with older adults. This is especially true as we start to employ more sensitive diagnostic tools. For example, the newer automated periodontal probes can measure much smaller changes in attachment loss than is possible using manual probes. It is conceivable that, at some point, if our only diagnostics are minute changes in attachment level, we may be measuring normal aging changes instead of active disease.

The loss of function of an organ system does not become significant until it crosses a given level. The functional performance of an organ in an elderly person depends on two principal factors: (1) the rate of deterioration (which varies greatly between individuals) and (2) the level of performance needed.[9] Most elderly people will have normal laboratory values. However, the critical difference, in fact the hallmark of aging, lies not in the resting level of performance but in how the organ adapts to external stress. For example, an older person may show a normal blood sugar at rest but be unable to handle a glucose load within the normal parameters for younger people, or an older person may have a normal resting pulse but be unable to achieve an adequate increase in cardiac output with exercise.

One thing to remember here is that most data come from cross-sectional (prevalence) studies in which individuals of different ages are compared in terms of group averages. Such an approach generally reveals a gradual decline. A few studies have followed cohorts of people longitudinally as they age. Their conclusions are quite different. For example, cognitive function can improve over time among older people and cardiac function in subjects free of heart disease does not show inevitable decline with age. The best predictor of a given person's performance now is the person's earlier performance rather than the average age-related decline.

II. Prevalence of Periodontal Diseases

Prevalence data from cross-sectional studies serve a number of purposes. These data are used to monitor the amount of disease existing in a population, to delineate the characteristics of people who have the disease, to generate hypotheses regarding the etiology of the disease, to plan manpower needs for preventive and treatment services, and to plan teaching programs. A series of properly conducted prevalence studies over time can be used to monitor trends in disease, effectiveness of preventive and treatment programs, and under certain conditions, to estimate incidence rates of disease. Thus, the data from these studies often are considered important and eagerly awaited by scientists, educators, and administrators.

Prevalence Related to Age

As will be the case for all the summary tables to be presented, there were a number of additional studies that made significant contributions to the literature that are not included, because the manner in which the data were presented did not readily allow appropriate comparisons. Table 1 presents findings from nine studies reporting the prevalence of periodontitis by age group. These studies were conducted in different countries on a wide variety of population groups and used a variety of methods to quantify disease. All of these studies indicated that the prevalence of pocket depth and attachment loss is higher in older age groups and that the prevalence of attachment loss is higher than the prevalence of pocket depth. One also is impressed by the effect of the definition of a "case" (e.g., 4mm, 6mm, 7mm) on the prevalences found. When the criterion of 4+mm of pocket depth are used as a definition of a case as compared with 6+mm, studies report prevalences of disease ranging from two to eight times higher with younger groups showing greater differences in prevalence than older groups. A similar pattern is seen for attachment loss.

Table 1 — Prevalence of Periodontitis in Various Age Groups

Study/Year	Measure	Age Range	Prevalences	Comments
NIDR,[10] 1986.	AL≥ 2mm PD≥ 4mm AL≥ 2mm AL≥ 4mm AL≥ 6mm PD≥ 4mm PD≥ 6mm	18-19, 60-64 18-19, 60-64 <65-65+ <65-65+ <65-65+ <65-65+ <65-65+	52%-95% 6%-24% 77%-95% 24%-68% +8%-34% 14%-22% +2%-4%	United States. Sample of working adults and sample of seniors attending senior centres. Half-mouth, 2 sites/tooth.
Brown et al.,[11] 1989.	PD>4mm PD>6mm	19-44, 45-64, 65+ 19-44, 45-64, 65+	25%-31%-34% 3%-16%-14%	United States, community-dwelling, collected 1981, 1 site/tooth.
Ismail et al.,[12] 1986.	PD 4-6mm PD 6+mm	27-46, 47-74 27-46, 47-74	34%-44% 8%-21%	2 New Mexico towns, normal and high F Six Ramfjord teeth, 2 sites/tooth.
Ismail et al.,[13] 1987.	AL 4-6mm AL 7+mm AL 4-6mm AL 7+mm	27-46, 47-74 27-46, 47-74 27-46 (1954) 27-46 (1954)	32%-72% 8%-32% 49% 14%	New Mexico in 1958, PDI and 2 New Mexico towns in 1984, see above.
Hoover & Tynan,[14] 1986.	AL >3 PD >5mm	19-29, 30-45, >45 19-29, 30-45, >45	8%-36%-72% 12%-11%-11%	Saskatoon, Canada. 4 surfaces of 6 teeth.
Papapanou et al.,[15] 1990.	PD≥4mm PD 6+mm	31-35, 61-65 31-35, 61-65	23%-29% 1.7%-5.3%	Random sample of Swedish industrial population. Six sites/tooth.* Pockets must also bleed.
Haikel et al.,[16] 1989.	PD 3.5-5.5 PD 6+mm	16-20, 41-60 16-20, 41-60	18.8%-54.6% 6.4%-34.1%	2 cities in Morocco. Sample of schools and health centres. Used CPITN on 6 teeth.
Miyazaki et al.,[17] 1989.	PD 4 or 5 PD 6+	15-19, 45-64 15-19, 45-64	6%-37% 0%-21%	National sample of Japan. Used CPITN.
Bergstrom and Eliasson[5] 1989.	PD 6+mm	21-30, 51-60	4%-43%	Sample of prof. musicians. Sweden. Dentally aware subjects, 6 sites/tooth.

Table 2 provides an opportunity for a closer comparison of prevalence rates for periodontal pocketing of 6 or more mm in middle aged adults. The six studies summarized in Table 2 report that between 11 percent and 43 percent of middle aged adults have one or more periodontal pockets measuring 6 or more millimetres. Thus all the studies indicate that the condition is present in a minority of the population. While the range of prevalences reported appears to be large, there appear to be handy explanations for the diversity of findings. The Brown et al.[11] and the Hoover and Tynan[14] studies, which reported the lowest prevalences, measured disease on only one site per tooth or used index teeth. These methods are known to underestimate the prevalence of the more serious levels of disease. The Ismail et al.[12] study also used index teeth, but included older individuals in their age groupings. Bergstrom and Eliasson[5] reported a prevalence of 43 percent in their 51-60 year age group. However, if this age group were to be combined with the younger age group to make them more comparable to the other studies, the overall prevalence would be more in the range shown in the other studies. Since the Bergstrom and Eliasson study population of professional musicians was characterized as "dentally aware", yet had generally higher prevalences than the other studies reported, higher prevalence may be due to using a probe graduated at 2mm increments or perhaps to some type of occupational risk. The two studies using the CPITN reported prevalence rates comparable to the other studies. The Haikel et al. study,[16] which reported the highest overall prevalence rate, sampled health centres for people who were not periodontal patients. However, this may have been a population in more frail health than in the other studies.

Table 2 — Prevalence of Middle Aged Adults
With One or More Periodontal Pockets of 6+ mm

Study/year	Age Group	Prevalence	Comments
Brown et al.,[11] 1989	45-64	16%	1 site/tooth
Ismail et al.,[12] 1986	45-79	21%	6 index teeth
Hoover & Tynan,[14] 1986	45+	11%	4 sur of 6 teeth
Bergstrom & Eliasson,[5] 1989	41-50, 51-60	22%, 43%	6 sur/tooth
Haikel et al.,[16] 1989	41-60	34%	CPITN
Miyazaki et al.,[17] 1989	45-64	21%	CPITN

Prevalence in Older Adults

Table 3 presents the prevalence of periodontal diseases in older adults in terms of the criterion used to define a "case". If periodontal disease is defined as one or more sites of attachment loss of 4 or more millimetres, then the vast majority of older adults have evidence of the disease. If periodontal disease is defined as one or more sites of attachment loss of 6 or more millimetres, then the condition appears to occur in less than half of the population. The exception is for blacks in North Carolina reported by Beck et al.[19] and potential reasons for this difference will be discussed later. Similar patterns are observed for the prevalence of periodontal disease measured in terms of pocket depth.

Two additional points not shown in Table 3 should be mentioned. First, most of these studies in both middle age and older adults show that the extent of the condition (number of sites in the mouth with the condition) is negatively associated with the severity of the definition of a "case", i.e., there are fewer sites in the mouth with 6mm pockets than with 4mm pockets. Thus, conditions of lower prevalence in the population also tend to have fewer sites involved. Second, most studies of people over age 65 that report the prevalence of disease by age group find that the prevalences are higher in the 65-69 and 70-74 year age groups than in the oldest age groups. These differences usually are attributed to the older age groups having lost more teeth. Thus, when thinking about the prevalence of disease in older adults, one always should consider the problem of tooth loss.

The Problem of Missing Teeth

The number of missing teeth also has implications for how seriously epidemiologic measures underestimate disease. Recent estimates of tooth loss due to periodontal disease are lower than the old conventional wisdom that after the age of 35 three-quarters of teeth lost are lost to periodontal disease. However, periodontal disease is responsible for a substantial amount of tooth loss in the population and may be the major cause of tooth loss in high risk individuals.[23-27] Thus, the prevalence of periodontal disease in older adults is likely to be an underestimate of the *periodontal disease experience* of the group and the degree of underestimation is likely to be a function of the number of teeth lost. However, the prevalence of pocket depths or attachment loss in a properly conducted study of an older population is likely to be an accurate estimate of the true prevalence of those conditions *during the period of time those measures were made*. Similarly, the change in attachment level is not likely to be affected by tooth loss, if the reason for tooth loss is ascertained.

Table 3 — Prevalence of Periodontal Diseases in Older Adults

Measure	Prevalence	Study/Year/Comments
AL≥4mm	68%	NIDR,[10] 1986, U.S. National Sample, Half-mouth, Senior Centres 2 sites/tooth.
	75%	Hunt et al.,[18] 2 Counties in Iowa, Community-dwelling 2 sites/tooth, full mouth.
	Whites 80% Blacks 91%	Beck et al.,[19] 1990. 5 Counties in North Carolina Community-dwelling, 2 sites/tooth, full mouth.
AL≥6mm	34%	NIDR,[10] 1986.
	30%	Hunt et al..[18]
	Whites 42% Blacks 71%	Beck et al.,[19] 1990.
	60%*	Yoneyama et al.,[20] 1988. Older cohorts from population from Ushiku, Japan. Full mouth. 6 sites/tooth. * Estimated from graph.
PD≥4mm	22%	NIDR,[10] 1986.
	34%	Brown et al.,[11] 1989, U.S. National sample, collected in 1981, community-dwelling, 1 site/tooth.
	Whites 34% Blacks 73%	Beck et al.,[19] 1990.
PD≥6mm	4%	NIDR,[10] 1986.
	Whites 10% Blacks 32%	Beck et al.,[21] 1988.
	14%	Brown et al.,[11] 1989.
	19-35%	Hu et al.,[22] 1990. Shanghai, China, CPITN Rates highest in 75-79 age group, 80+ group had lowest prevalence and lowest number of teeth.

On the other hand, the lack of a measure of whether disease is active in a site could result in epidemiologic data over-estimating the prevalence of disease. The use of "change in the level of attachment" as a measure in longitudinal studies makes this less of a concern with incidence studies using comparable definitions of a "case."

Indicators of Risk for Periodontitis

As stated above, characteristics identified in prevalence studies (cross-sectional studies) that are associated with people having higher odds of disease are more properly referred to as risk indicators rather than as risk factors. This is because prevalence studies can only describe associations evident at a point in time and cannot determine that one event preceded the other.

Before discussing the characteristics that have been associated with periodontitis, it is helpful to illustrate the process by which risk indicators (and for incidence studies, risk factors) can be identified and what some of those indicators might be. For this illustration, I will present some published data from the Piedmont 65+ Dental Study[19] and additional unpublished findings on microorganisms.

The prevalence of deep pockets and severe loss of attachment in the Piedmont 65+ sample has already been presented and implies that older blacks have a much higher prevalence of disease than older whites. As in other studies, we found a higher prevalence of disease than in younger populations, and there appeared to be a small group of people with most of the serious disease. Thus, further analyses are needed to focus on two questions: 1) What were the characteristics that differentiated the people with serious disease from the others, and 2) Were any of these characteristics different for blacks and whites? Since attachment loss and pocketing were prevalent in these older adults, but generally not severe, we needed to come up with a definition of a "case" of serious periodontitis in this older population that would be mindful of the distribution of disease in this population and, at the same time, clinically relevant. After consultation with a number of clinical periodontists, we arrived at a definition of disease that most clinicians felt was of concern. Thus, serious periodontal disease was defined as having four or more sites with loss of attachment of 5 or more millimetres and one or more of those sites had a pocket depth of 4 or more millimetres. This definition resulted in 46% of blacks and 16% of whites having a serious periodontal condition. Table 4 presents the characteristics associated with serious disease for blacks. Oral factors associated with serious disease were having greater than 2% *Prevotella intermedia* and greater than 2% *Porphyromonas gingivalis* in plaque samples, and gums having bled during the last 2 weeks when brushing or for no apparent reason. Social or background factors were having less than a high school education, below average socio-economic status, and the money available not meeting basic needs. Behavioural factors were the use of tobacco and not having been to the dentist in the last 3 years. Finally, an apparent physical indicator, morning cough, is associated with serious disease. Risk indicators for whites were similar. Thus, a large number of risk indicators were identified because certain characteristics were associated with our definition of serious disease in older adults. However, some of these characteristics could be associated with serious disease because they are associated with another characteristic. For example, morning cough may be associated with serious disease because it is associated with the use of tobacco products, which are associated with serious disease. In order to determine the relative strength of the associations already identified, a multivariate analysis was conducted.

Table 4[*] — Odds of Black Respondents having Four or More Sites with Loss of Attachment of 5+mm and One or More of those Sites Having a Pocket Depth of 4+ mm for Selected Factors: Piedmont 65+ Dental Study, 1988

Indicator	Odds Ratio	95% Confidence Bound	Significance
Education <12 vs 12+	3.1	1.639 — 6.029	<0.001
Use Tob vs No Use	2.8	1.712 — 4.697	<0.001
Gums Bleed Last 2 Weeks (Yes vs No)	3.2	1.793 — 5.797	<0.001
Last Visit to the Dentist (>3 Years vs <3 Years)	2.7	1.631 — 4.428	<0.001
P. Intermeda (>2% vs 2% or Less)	1.9	1.129 — 3.100	0.015
P. gingivalis (>2% vs 2% or Less)	2.7	1.459 — 4.932	0.001
Duncan SES Index (Below Median vs Above)	1.7	1.017 — 2.761	0.043
Morning Cough (Yes vs No)	2.2	1.075 — 4.493	0.028
How Well does Money Meet Needs (Poorly vs Other)	2.0	1.081 — 3.558	0.026

[*] Source: Beck et al.,[19] 1990.

Table 5* — Logistic Model for Blacks having 4+ Sites of Attachment loss of 5+mm and One or More of those Sites Having a Pocket of 4+ mm: Piedmont 65+ Dental Study, 1988

Variable	Beta	Odds Ratio	95% Confidence Bound	Level of Significance
Intercept	-1.7299			<0.001
Tobacco Use (0=No 1=Use)	1.0588	2.8829	1.6145 — 5.1478	<0.001
P. gingivalis (0= ≤2%, 1= >2%)	0.8800	2.4109	1.2330 — 4.7139	0.010
P. intermedia (0= ≤2%, 1= >2%)	0.6202	1.8593	1.7686 — 1.9547	0.033
Last Visit to the Dentist (0= ≤3 Years, 1= >3 Years)	0.8207	2.2721	1.2893 — 4.0042	0.004
Gums Bleed Last 2 Weeks (0=No, 1=Yes)	1.3511	3.8617	1.9875 — 7.5033	<0.001

Percent Correctly Classified   = 70.7
Sensitivity   = 63.5
Specificity   = 77.1
* Source: Beck et al.,[19] 1990.

Table 5 presents the model for blacks, which contains only main effects. The characteristic with the strongest association with serious disease was an interview item on whether their gums had bled in the last 2 weeks either when brushing or for no apparent reason. People who responded "yes" had almost 4 times the odds of having serious disease. People with greater than 2% *P. gingivalis* or *P. intermedia* had 2.4 or 1.9 times the odds respectively. Finally, people whose last visit to the dentist was more than 3 years ago had approximately 2.3 times the odds of having serious disease. People having all of the characteristics in the model would have 113 times the odds of having a serious periodontal condition than people who had none of the characteristics. As very few people had all the characteristics, a less stringent rule of having any four of the five characteristics would result in their having 14 times the odds for a serious periodontal condition. Since microorganisms, using tobacco, and not visiting the dentist regularly were the important risk indicators for whites also, we looked further into the role of microorganisms. As shown in Table 6, attachment loss of 7 or more millimetres occurred in 11.6% of blacks and 3.1% of whites. Sites experiencing attachment loss of 5+ and 7+ mm were approximately three times more prevalent in blacks. Thus, blacks were more likely to experience attachment loss of 5+ or 7+ mm and more sites were affected. *Actinobacillus actinomycetemcomitans* and *P. intermedia* were twice as likely to be found in sites of blacks than in sites of whites. The most striking contrasts between blacks and whites appeared as four-fold differences in the prevalence of *P. gingivalis* and six-fold differences in the number of sites with this organism.

Table 6 — Prevalence of Clinical and Microbiological Variables for 366 Black and 297 White Piedmont 65+ Respondents

	Percent of Sites* with Condition for:		Percent of Subjects* with Condition for:	
	Blacks	Whites	Blacks	Whites
Attachment Loss (AL) AL of 7+mm	11.6 (1.1)	3.1 (0.5)	54.3 (2.8)	27.6 (2.8)
Pocket Depth 6+mm	44.4 (0.6)	0.7 (0.1)	32.1 (2.7)	9.8 (1.9)
P. intermedia	30.0 (1.8)	14.6 (1.6)	55.6 (2.9)	33.1 (3.0)
P. gingivalis	18.6 (1.7)	3.4 (0.7)	39.0 (3.1)	9.4 (1.9)

* Standard error in parentheses.

Table 7 presents the relationship between the presence of *P. gingivalis* and the prevalence of sites with loss of attachment of 7+mm, considering the lack of independence of sites within each person for blacks and whites. In the first comparison, blacks with *P. gingivalis* present have 2.7 times more sites with LA of 7+ mm than blacks without *P. gingivalis*. Similarly, whites with *P. gingivalis* present have 3 times more sites with LA of 7+ mm. The prevalence of sites with LA of 7+ mm is higher for blacks than whites when both have *P. gingivalis* absent. When *P. gingivalis* is present in both blacks and whites, the tendency for higher prevalence of sites with LA of 7+ mm in blacks is suggestive but not significantly greater. Similar analyses for the relationships between *P. gingivalis* and pocket depths greater than 6mm and *P. intermedia* and loss of attachment and pocket depth produced identical results.

Table 7 — Relationships between Presence of *P. gingivalis* and Prevalence of Sites with Loss of Attachment, Considering Lack of Independence within Each Person and Weighted at the Patient Level

Group	Prevalence of Sites with LA of 7+mm	Prevalence Ratios	Confidence Intervals	Survey-based p
Blacks: Pg+	0.289	2.77	1.97 — 3.88	0.000
Blacks: Pg-	0.107			
Whites: Pg+	0.133	3.04	1.21 — 7.66	0.018
Whites: Pg-	0.044			
Blacks: Pg+	0.298	2.23	0.95 — 5.27	0.067
Whites: Pg+	0.133			
Blacks: Pg-	0.107	2.45	1.58 — 3.81	0.000
Whites: Pg-	0.044			
Homogeneity				0.850

The preceding analyses indicated that *P. gingivalis* explains some of the differences in the prevalence of loss of attachment and pocket depth within each race and between each race. However, when *P. gingivalis* is absent, blacks have a higher prevalence of disease than whites. To look for other factors that may account for the racial differences in attachment loss observed in this population, a logistic regression model was developed for loss of attachment of 7+ mm that excluded race. This model, presented in Table 8, indicates that the presence of *P. gingivalis*, having few teeth, having visited the dentist more than 3 years ago, having *P. intermedia* present, and using tobacco were associated with attachment loss of 7+ mm. Furthermore, when race was added to this model it no longer was significant, indicating that these variables explained most of the differences seen in attachment loss between blacks and whites. These analyses indicate that some of the difference in the prevalence of severe disease between blacks and whites can be explained by the different prevalences of *P. gingivalis* and *P. intermedia.* However, these microorganisms do not explain all of the differences. For example, when *P. gingivalis* is absent, blacks still have higher prevalences of disease than whites. In addition, when these microorganisms are present, a higher proportion of sites in blacks have indications of severe disease. Hence, it may be necessary to look at other factors to account for racial differences in attachment loss more fully. Explanatory variables that were not measured in this study, such as factors related to host response and additional microorganisms, such as *Bacteroides forsythus, Fusobacterium nucleatum, Wolinella recta, Eikenella corrodens,* and spirochetes could account for some of the difference in the prevalence of attachment loss and pocket depth between blacks and whites. In addition to *P. gingivalis* and *P. intermedia,* nonbacterial factors such as having visited a dentist more than three years ago, having few teeth, and using tobacco were significant in the logistic regression model for having attachment loss of 7mm or greater. It is noteworthy that once the above explanatory variables are accounted for in the model, race is no longer a significant explanatory variable. This may indicate that behaviours related to use of dental services and use of tobacco as well as aspects related to infection rates and host response may be fruitful areas of future investigation for identification of risk factors.

Table 8 — Stepwise Logistic Regression Model for Loss of Attachment of 7+mm: Piedmont 65+ Dental Study, 1988

Variable	Beta	Odds Ratio	95% Confidence Bound
Intercept	-0.5086		
Pg (1=present)	0.9285	2.5	2.036 — 3.024
Number of Teeth	-0.0517	0.9	0.913 — 0.966
Last Visit to the Dentist (1=>3 Years)	0.6995	2.0	1.602 — 2.418
Pi (1=present)	0.6172	1.9	1.419 — 2.281
Tobacco (1=use)	0.5437	1.7	1.296 — 2.144
Race	Not significant		

Total odds = 16.2

With the above illustration of how risk indicators can be identified in epidemiologic studies, Table 9 presents characteristics that have been associated with the prevalence of periodontitis in studies that used multivariate analyses. These characteristics appear to be associated with periodontitis, adjusting for other characteristics in the model. Since the different studies did not always include the same characteristics in their models, each of the indicators in this table should not be considered to be related to pocket depth or attachment loss, adjusting for all of the other characteristics in the table.

Table 9 — Multi-variate Associations Between Risk Indicators and Prevalence of Periodontitis

Indicator	Pocket Depth			Loss of Attachment		
	Number Studies	Positive Assoc.	Negative Assoc.	Number Studies	Positive Assoc.	Negative Assoc.
Age group	1	1		3	2	
Race	1			2	2	
Education	1			2		
Sex	1			2		
Dental Visits				1	1	
Finances				1		
Tobacco				2	2	
Alcohol				1	1	
Cognition				1		
Hypertension				1	1	
Stress				1		1
Social Particip.				1		1
No. Teeth				1		1
Coronal Caries				1		
Root Caries				2	1	
Microorganisms				1	1	
Calculus				2	1	
Teeth w Plaque	1	1		2	1	
Sites w Bleeding	1			1		

It is obvious that only a few studies have analyzed data in a multivariate manner. Thus, most of the risk indicators that have be identified could be associated with each other. Only one study reviewed showed that being older was associated with a greater prevalence of deep pockets while controlling for other characteristics. Likewise, a similar relationship was found for plaque in one study. Education level, sex, race, and number of sites with bleeding were found not to be associated with prevalence of deep pockets. The use of the remaining indicators has not been reported in relation to pocket depth. In the three studies that analyzed age in relation to loss of attachment, two found that being older was associated with a higher prevalence of loss of attachment. Similarly, race and use of tobacco have been found to be associated with loss of attachment in two studies. Other indicators found to be associated with loss of attachment in a single study included frequency of dental visits, alcohol use, hypertension, stress, lack of social participation, having few teeth, the presence of micro-organisms, root caries, calculus, and number of teeth with plaque. On the other hand, education level and sex were included in the analyses in two studies and neither study found them to be associated.

III. Incidence of Periodontal Diseases

Incidence Studies

Since longitudinal studies are more complex to design, take longer to complete, and are more expensive to conduct, it is not surprising that only a few studies reporting changes in the level of attachment loss in populations have been reported in the last five years. The incidence of attachment loss (loss of attachment over time) found in four studies is summarized in Table 10. Like the prevalence studies, these incidence studies were conducted on widely varying populations using different definitions of a "case". Furthermore, these studies vary in length from one to twenty-eight years.

The Löe et al.[28] study reports on the incidence of attachment loss in a group of tea workers in Sri Lanka. In this population that had little or no oral care, about 8 percent of the group experienced rapid periodontal destruction with major tooth loss, about 81 percent had moderate destruction, and about 11 percent experienced minimal or no disease. In populations that appear to have received home and professional care, the incidence of attachment loss was much less dramatic and appeared primarily to be confined to a small high risk group. In the other studies summarized in Table 10, most of the groups experiencing attachment loss comprised from 5 to 43 percent of the population. Again, the size of the high risk groups varied according to the definition of disease and characteristics of the study populations. The Levy et al.[29] study produced the only data confined to older adults. They defined disease progression as two or more sites which experienced two or more millimetres of attachment loss over a two year period and found the incidence to be 17 percent. Ismail et al.[30] re-examined a population originally studied in 1959 and found that the incidence of disease was higher in older cohorts that younger cohorts.

Table 10 — Proportion of Population with Incidence of Attachment Loss

Study	Measure	Proportion	Time	Comment
Löe et al.[28] 1986	Before age 21 4+mm on 2+ molars or inc. or before 30 8 Missing T or w LA 5+mm	8%	15 yrs	Little or no oral care. 14-46 years of age. 480 male tea workers in Sri Lanka.
Levy et al.[29] 1990	2+ sites with 2+ mm AL	17%	2 yrs	Over age 70, Community-dwelling 2 Iowa counties, full-mouth, 2 sites/tooth.
	Mean Increase ≥ 0.2mm	20%		
	Mean Increase ≥ 0.4mm	7%		
Ismail et al.[30] 1990	*Mean Increase ≥ 2.0mm*		28 yrs	Same population of Tecumseh, Mich. examined in 1959 and 1987. N=167. 4 sites/tooth, full-mouth, ages 31-87.
	Born 1900-24	23%		
	Born 1925-34	17%		
	Born 1935-44	17%		
	Born 1945-54	5%		
Haffajee et al.[31] 1991	*AL of 3+mm @ 1+ sites*		1 yr	271 samples in Ushiku, Japan age 20+, full-mouth, 6 sites/tooth.
	40-49	31%		
	50-59	32%		
	>59	43%		

This has been a consistent finding in most longitudinal studies. Using a definition of a mean increase in attachment loss of 2 or more millimetres (the most conservative definition of a case in this group of studies), they found an incidence of disease in middle-aged cohorts of 17 percent and an incidence of 23 percent in the oldest cohorts who were between 64 and 87 years old. Because Ismail et al.[30] required a greater level of periodontal destruction to be considered a case than did Levy et al.,[29] it is not possible to compare the rates.

However, if one were to speculate that the differences in the duration of the studies cancelled out the differences in the definition of a case, then the incidence rates do seem to be similar. Haffajee et al.[31] found rates reaching 43 percent in a one-year study of a population in Japan. Reasons for the high rates may be the characteristics of the population examined and examining six sites per tooth.

Risk Factors/Predictors of Attachment Loss

Characteristics that have been looked at as possible risk factors or predictors of attachment loss are presented in Table 11. In this instance, the difference between a risk factor and a predictor is that risk factors are thought to be causal. Although both bivariate and multivariate associations are presented for completeness, only multivariate associations will be discussed. All three studies that considered age found that being older was associated with a higher incidence of attachment loss. The only other characteristics associated with incidence of attachment loss more than once were the percent of sites with recession greater than 1mm and having only a few teeth. It is not clear whether any of these characteristics are risk factors or simply good predictors of attachment loss. Other characteristics that have been associated with incidence of attachment loss are birth cohort (when they were born), being male, smoking, and tooth type. Other characteristics that most likely are predictors rather than risk factors are percent of sites with gingivitis at baseline, mean attachment loss at baseline, and percent of baseline sites with pocket depths greater than 3mm.

Table 11 — Risk Factors for Attachment Loss

Indicator	Bi-variate			Multi-variate		
	Number Studies	Positive Assoc.	Negative Assoc.	Number Studies	Positive Assoc.	Negative Assoc.
Birth Cohort	1	1		1	1	
Age Group	3	3		3	3	
Age Group (65+)	1					
Sex	3			1	1	
Xerostomic Meds.	1	1				
Smoking	3	3		1	1	

Table 11 — Risk Factors for Attachment Loss

Indicator	Bi-variate			Multi-variate		
	Number Studies	Positive Assoc.	Negative Assoc.	Number Studies	Positive Assoc.	Negative Assoc.
Health Status Poor	1	1				
Diabetes	1	1				
Education	1	1				
Dental Visits	1	1				
Have Insurance	1	1				
Income	1					
Perceived Need Visit	1	1				
Tooth Mobility	1	1		1	1	
No. Missing Teeth	3		1	2		2
% Sites w Gingivitis	1			1		
% Sites w Plaque	3	2		1		
Bleed on Probing	1	1		1		
Mean Baseline PD	1	1		1		
Mean Baseline AL	1	1		2	1	
% Sites AL>3mm	2	2		1		
% Sites PD>3mm	1	1		1	1	
% Sites Rec>1mm	1	1		2	2	
Oral Hygiene Index	1	1				
Root Caries Experience	1	1				
Tooth Type				1	1	

IV. Discussion and Conclusions

I have approached the assigned topic, the epidemiology of periodontal diseases in older adults with emphasis on risk factors, in a very simplistic manner. Historically, few epidemiologic studies have addressed the problem of periodontitis in older adults and some of those have used indices that are not directly comparable with recent studies. Thus, this review has been restricted to studies reported in the last five years. In addition, I have attempted to reduce this complex entity, periodontitis, to two questions. The first question was, What is the prevalence (defined as the percent of people with periodontal pockets or attachment loss) and incidence (defined as the percent of people with a change in attachment loss over a period of time) in the population? The second question was, What are possible risk indicators (defined as characteristics associated with prevalence of periodontal pockets and attachment loss) and risk factors (defined as characteristics associated with the incidence of attachment loss) for periodontitis? The correct answer to the first question is that the prevalence and incidence of periodontitis depends on what definition of "a case" was used in the study and the measurement techniques that were used. The variety of definitions and methods used make it difficult to draw any firm conclusions. Thus, some infirm conclusions follow:

1. Most studies agree that the prevalence and incidence of periodontitis increases in middle-age and older cohorts. In fact, the studies reviewed on the prevalence of pocket depths of 6+mm indicate that middle-aged and older adults may have comparable prevalences. However, the incidence studies seem to indicate that the incidence of attachment loss is greater in older adults, implying that differential rates of tooth loss are affecting the prevalence estimates for the two age groups.

2. In older adults, the prevalences of attachment loss > 4mm (68-91%) appear to be approximately twice as high as the prevalences of attachment loss of > 6mm (30-71%). However, the implications for treatment needs in older adults are not as clear as if this were a younger cohort.

3. Considering the diversity of definitions of "a case", study length, and methods used in the few incidence studies reported, the findings are surprisingly similar. The incidence of attachment loss in the middle-age and older cohorts in the studies reviewed appear to involve between 17 and 43 percent of the people, with the higher rates

reported in the Japanese study. These rates appear to be higher than rates usually reported for younger cohorts.

The answer to the second question must be the same as the answer to the first question, because risk factors for a disease can vary with the definition of a "case". In addition, we should not assume that risk factors for a disease operate consistently for older and younger people and, consequently, we should not assume the risk factors or a risk model for periodontal disease in younger people will work equally as well for older people. However, a few trends seem apparent from the small number of studies that have used multivariate analyses to identify risk factors/predictors.

1. There are a wide variety of characteristics that appear to precede the incidence of attachment loss. These characteristics are oral, socio-economic, demographic, medical, and behavioural in nature and verify the potentially complex nature of periodontitis. Age group, number of missing teeth, and the percent of sites with recession >1mm have been identified by more than one study. While these characteristics may be good predictors of future attachment loss, it is unlikely that any of these predictors are causal and, therefore, risk factors. In fact, the majority of the oral characteristics identified probably are risk predictors rather than risk factors. The finding that birth cohort is a significant predictor has potentially important implications for the rates of periodontitis than we might expect as younger cohorts age and this finding should be explored more fully.

2. Characteristics such as smoking, diabetes, and dental visits have been found to precede attachment loss in bivariate analyses. These relationships provide support for a number of clinical studies and studies of specific population groups that have found these to be risk factors (32-38). It is unfortunate that studies employing multivariate analyses using these risk factors have not been conducted.

While making firm conclusions regarding the prevalence, incidence, and risk factors/predictors for periodontitis in older adults would be risky, some patterns have emerged. In addition, this attempt to present the epidemiology of periodontitis clarified some directions for future endeavours.

First, some consensus on the definition of a "case" of disease is desperately needed. It is virtually impossible to compare the prevalence or incidence of disease in different populations when there is no consensus about what is disease. If a single case definition is not appropriate, then some consensus should be reached on definitions of a "case" in certain population groups, e.g., older adults versus younger that could be used. We should remember that the "case" definition in most instances does not affect how the condition is measured, but simply involves a re-analysis of the data already collected. With some measure of consistency in a definition, much additional information on the prevalence and incidence of disease could be gleaned from re-analyses. In addition, either a consensus on measurement techniques employed in studies is needed, or correction factors when using partial recording methods must be determined and used.

Second, there were many articles reviewed that provided a great deal of useful information about patterns of disease within the mouth or presented only mean scores that could have provided more basic prevalence and incidence information. Thus, there really is more information available that could not be used in this type of review. It would be useful if authors could provide basic prevalence and incidence findings along with their other analyses.

Third, it is conceptually useful to distinguish between risk indicators and risk factors and between risk factors and risk predictors. Some clarity in our "risk prediction language" can only enhance our efforts.

Fourth, some longitudinal studies are still being conducted that do not make use of multivariate analysis techniques to determine the importance of risk factors/predictors while accounting for the effect of the other factors. Thus, some of our current information on risk factors could be updated through additional analyses of available data.

Last, it is obvious that, currently, a large number of potential risk factors for periodontitis have been identified in epidemiologic studies. In addition, there are putative risk factors that have not been verified in epidemiologic studies, e.g., microorganisms, in combination with other risk factors. We are in need of population-based studies that can evaluate the relative contributions of a variety of possible risk factors, including markers of infection and host response.

Endnotes

1.   Koch GG, Beck JD. Statistical concepts: a matrix for identification of model types. In: Bader JD. *Risk assessment in dentistry.* Chapel Hill: University of North Carolina Dental Ecology, 1990:174-92.

2.   Beck JD. Identification of risk factors. In: Bader JD. *Risk assessment in dentistry.* Chapel Hill: University of North Carolina Dental Ecology, 1990:8-13.

3.   Lilienfeld AM. *Foundations of epidemiology.* New York: Oxford University Press, 1976; 255-62.

4.   Russell AL. A system of classification and scoring for prevalence surveys of periodontal disease. *J Dent Res.* 1956;35:350-9.

5.   Bergstrom J, Eliasson S. Prevalence of chronic periodontal disease using probing depth as a diagnostic test. *J Clin Periodontal.* 1989; 16:588-92.

6.   Goodson JM. Selection of suitable indicators of periodontitis. In: Bader JD. *Risk assessment in dentistry.* Chapel Hill: University of North Carolina Dental Ecology, 1990:69-74.

7.   Clark WB, Magnusson I. Field measurement of risk factors for periodontitis. In: Bader JD. *Risk assessment in dentistry.* Chapel Hill: University of North Carolina Dental Ecology, 1990:225-33.

8.   Ainamo J, Barmes D, Beagrie G, Cutress T, Martin J, Sardo-Infirri J. Development of the World Health Organization (WHO) community periodontal index of treatment needs (CPITN). *Int Dent J.* 1982; 32:281-91.

9.   Kane RL, Ouslander JG, Abrass IB. *Essentials of clinical geriatrics.* Second edition. New York: McGraw-Hill. 1989.

10.   U.S. Department of Health and Human Services. Oral health of United States adults: The national survey of oral health in U.S. employed adults and seniors, 1985-1986. Bethesda, Maryland: National Institute of Dental Research; 1987; *NIH Publication.* No. 87-2868.

11.   Brown LJ, Oliver RC, Loe H. Periodontal diseases in the U.S. in 1981: prevalence, severity, extent, and role in tooth mortality. *J. Periodontal.* 1989;60:363-70.

12.   Ismail AI, Eklund SA, Burt BA, Calderone JJ. Prevalence of deep periodontal pockets in New Mexico adults aged 27-74 years. *J Public Health Dent.* 1986; 46(4):199-206.

13.   Ismail AI, Eklund SA, Striffler DF, Szpunar SM. The prevalence of advanced loss of periodontal attachment in two New Mexico populations. *J Periodontal Res.* 1987; 22:119-24.

14. Hoover JN, Tynan JJ. Periodontal status of a group of Canadian adults. *J Canad Dent Assn*. 1986, No. 9:761-63.
15. Papananou PN, Wennstrom JL, Sellen A, Hirooka H, Grondahl K, Johnsson T. Periodontal treatment needs assessed by the use of clinical and radiographic criteria. *Community Dent Oral Epidemiol*. 1990; 18:113-9.
16. Haikel Y, Turlot J-C, Cahen P-M, Frank R. Periodontal treatment needs in populations of high- and low-fluoride areas of Morocco. *J Clin Periodontal*. 1989; 16:596-600.
17. Miyazaki H, et al. Periodontal disease prevalence in different age groups in Japan as assessed according to the CPITN. *Community Dent Oral Epidemiol*. 1989; 17:71-4.
18. Hunt RJ, Levy SM, Beck JD. The prevalence of periodontal attachment loss in an Iowa population aged 70 and older. *J Public Health Dent*. 1990; 50(4): 252-56.
19. Beck JD, Koch GG, Rozier RG, Tudor GE. Prevalence and risk indicators for periodontal attachment loss in a population of older community-dwelling blacks and whites. *J Periodontal*. 1990; 61:521-28.
20. Yoneyama T, Okamoto H, Lindhe J, Socransky SS, Haffajee AD. Probing depth, attachment loss and gingival recession. *J Clin Periodontal*. 1988; 15:581-91.
21. Beck JD, Koch GG. Pocket depth and attachment loss in community-dwelling older adults. *J Dent Res*. 1989; 68(Spec Issue):863.
22. Hu C-Z, Huang C-R, Rong S, Zhang W, Wu J, Pilot T. Periodontal conditions in elderly people of Shanghai, People's Republic of China, in 1986. *Community Dent Health*. 1990; 7:69-71.
23. Hand J, Hunt RJ, Kohout F. Five-year incidence of tooth loss in Iowans aged 65 and older. *Community Dent Oral Epidemiol*. (In press).
24. Bouma J, Schaub RMH, Poel ACM van de. Relative importance of periodontal disease for full mouth extractions in the Netherlands. *Community Dent Oral Epidemiol*. 1987; 15: 41-5.
25. Burt BA, Ismail AI, Morrison EC, Beltran ED. Risk factors for tooth loss over a 28-year period. *J Dent Res*. 1990; 69(5):1126-30.
26. Ainamo J, Sarkki L, Kuhalampi ML, Palolampi L, Piirto O. The frequency of periodontal extractions in Finland. 1984; 1:165-72.
27. Lindhe J, Okamoto H, Yoneyama T, Haffajee A, Socransky SS. Longitudinal changes in periodontal disease in untreated subjects. *J Clin Periodontal*. 1989; 16:662-70.

28. Löe H, Anerud A, Boysen H, Morrison E. Natural history of periodontal disease in man. Rapid, moderate and no loss of attachment in Sri Lankan labourers 14 to 46 years of age. *J Clin Periodontal*. 1986; 13:431-40.
29. Levy SM, Fann SJ, Kohout RJ. Factors related to the incidence of periodontal attachment loss. *J Dent Res*. 1990; 69(Special Issue): 211.
30. Ismail AI, Morrison EC, Burt BA, Caffesse RG, Kavanagh MT. Natural history of periodontal disease in adults: findings from the Tecumseh periodontal disease study, 1959-87. *J Dent Res*. 1990; 69(2):430-35.
31. Haffajee AD, Socransky SS, Lindhe J, Kent RL, Okamoto H, Yoneyama T. Clinical risk indicator for periodontal attachment loss. *J Clin Periodontal*. 1991;18:117-25.
32. Feldman RS, Alman JE, Chauncey HH. Periodontal disease indexes and tobacco smoking in healthy aging men. *Gerodontics*. 1987; 1:43-6.
33. Goultschin J, Sagan Cohen HD, Donchin M, Brayer L, Soskolne WA. Association of smoking with periodontal treatment needs. *J Periodontal*. 1990; 61:364-67.
34. Feldman RS, Bravacos JS, Rose CL. Association between smoking different tobacco products and periodontal disease indexes. *J. Periodontal*. 1983; 54:481-87.
35. Enrich LJ, Shlossman M, Genco RJ. Periodontal disease in non-insulin-dependent diabetes mellitus. *J Periodontal*. 1991; 62: 123-30.
36. Nelson RG, Shlossman M, Budding LM, et al. Periodontal disease in NIDDM in Pima Indians. *Diabetes Care*. 1990; 13:836-40.
37. Hugoson A, Thorstensson H, Falk H, Kuylenstierna J. Periodontal conditions in insulin-dependent diabetics. *J Clin Periodontal*. 1989; 16:215-23.
38. Hayden P, Buckley LA. Diabetes mellitus and periodontal disease in an Irish population. *J Periodont Res*. 1989; 24:298-302.

Chapter 3
Periodontal Services for Older Adults:
What They Need and What They Get

James L. Leake and David Locker

Introduction

I last stood on this platform 25 years ago as a new graduate. Thinking back on that event, in the context of today's presentation, I only wish I were now half as confident about anything as I was then, about everything. So please accept these remarks from one who is still questioning rather than from someone who is certain.

Statement of Problem

In Ontario we have no recent estimates of either the prevalence or the severity of periodontal disease in the adult population, nor how much care is currently provided by dentists and hygienists. The lack of such information, on the needs and adequacy of care for periodontal disease, is holding back development of public policy, curriculum revision and quality assurance in Ontario. For example, the Advisory Committee to the Minister of Health on Dental Care for Seniors in Need recommended that such data be gathered as part of the information needed to rationally plan a dental care program for seniors.[1] Similarly, university-based curriculum planners have not had information on which to justify revisions to either undergraduate or postgraduate curricula. Further, since formal quality assurance is soon to be mandated in Ontario, a knowledge of the public's need for, and the profession's current provision of, periodontal care would help in at least deciding the priority of quality assurance in this area. That is, if all needs were well addressed, then quality assurance might more profitably be directed to other areas.

Relevance of Study to the Problem

During 1988 and 1989 we surveyed adults aged 50 and over from four communities in Ontario. We gathered information in three stages: a telephone interview; a direct personal interview along with an epidemiologic examination of oral health status and need for care; and, lastly, a questionnaire mailed to named dental care providers on services provided. This data base on older adults offers the opportunity to examine the issues of disease prevalence, need for care and the methods by and the extent to which that need is addressed.

Literature Review

1. *Periodontal Status*

Capilouto and Douglass analyzed data from repeated national surveys in the United States.[2] They found that:

1) gingivitis has probably declined consistent with national trends towards improved oral hygiene, increased dental care utilization and decreased smoking, plus the use of antibiotics and increased use of fluorides;
2) periodontal disease appears to affect about 20 percent of the population, although severity, as measured by probing depths, may be declining; and
3) older groups continue to exhibit more disease than younger groups.

A 1989 report by Brown, Oliver and Löe[3] also showed that only 8% of all adults in the 1981 United States adult population had the most severe category of adult periodontitis. Among the elderly, only 14% of those aged 65+ had one or more pockets >6mm and nearly 52% had no pockets >4mm.

Hunt and others have conducted the most recent province-wide study of oral health in Ontario. They reported that, in 1978, the periodontal index scores of Ontario adults aged 35-44 were low compared to six other countries in the first ICS study.[4] Leake et al.[5] and Slade et al.[6] have reported on older Ontario adults living independently in East York and Ottawa-Carleton. They found between 9% and 21% of those over 50 and over 65 years had pockets of 6mm or deeper.

2. *Estimating Treatment Needs*

Estimating needs for care from epidemiologic data is difficult. *First,* the epidemiologic method requires that the condition be definitely present before it can be recorded.[7] *Second,* epidemiologic field measurements seldom record findings on all sites. Rather, the protocol defines standard sites to represent all. Thus, the epidemiologic method has an inherent bias to understate severity and perhaps prevalence levels compared to a full clinical assessment of all sites in an individual.[8] *Third,* dentists lack clinical indicators with which to accurately identify active periodontal disease,[9] although a recently developed test may be helpful in chairside monitoring of the presence of some bacteria often associated with disease.[10] *Fourth,* and perhaps as a consequence of the last point, there is, as yet, no ideal intervention to cure periodontal disease[11,12] and thus, dentists would be expected to vary since no one can state, with certainty, which of the array of possible interventions is needed.

The joint FDI/WHO Working Group[13] has classified the types of care needed to correspond to the CPITN scores as:

TN0 = no treatment required
TN1 = oral hygiene instruction
TN2 = scaling and prophylaxis + TN1
TN3 = complex treatment + TN2

Hunt defines the type of care according to CPITN scores as above but specifies root planing in sextants where CPITN = 3 and extraction where teeth are excessively mobile.[14]

Bader and others[15] estimated the time required for treatment of regular dental patients according to their CPITN sextant scores. They used time values derived empirically in an earlier study on dental practices in the United States.

Oliver, Brown and Löe[16] use evidence from randomized controlled trials to define current best treatment according to the person's periodontal scores. They then calculated times for each defined procedure per quadrant, weighted by the number of teeth in the quadrant. For some procedures, e.g., prophylaxis, they used times per individuals.

3. *What do Dentists Provide?*

Periodontal care makes up a minority of general dentists' services. Douglass and Furino[17] estimated that periodontal care represented only about 4.5% of general dental practice. This was confirmed by Grembowski, Milgrom and Fiset,[18] who have shown that, amid a great deal of variation, mean periodontal procedures made up only 2.6% of all services. This excludes prophylaxes, which were 25% of all services. Periodontal services were provided 14 times more frequently in dental practices with the highest expenditure per patient.

Looking at the issue from the perspective of the patient, an audit of 2488 5-year records of patients in 36 North Carolina general dental practices showed that only 16% of records had any indication of a periodontal diagnosis but 36% had indication of periodontal care.[19]

During the second (steady-state) year of the Rand study of dental insurance, Bailit and Manning[20] reported that between 2% to 3% of subjects received scaling, curettage or surgery. Forty-one percent received prophylaxis. Among subjects in poorest health (PI scores of 6 or 8), the probability of receiving prophylaxis was less than half (.22 vs. .55) that of the healthiest patients. The probability of this needy group getting scalings and curettage was .03. These data are consistent with Diehr and Grembowski's[21] findings of 23 scalings provided per 1000 patients in a Washington State teacher's group.

This low level of care provision occurs in spite of population-based estimates of need[22] and an historic perception among dentists that periodontal disease is both widely prevalent and the major cause of tooth loss in adults.[23]

4. Effectiveness of Current Care Levels

Conventional methods and levels of care do not appear to meet patients' needs. Periodontal disease indices persist at relatively high levels even among regular attenders. In a baseline assessment of 1092 patients in 36 North Carolina offices, 52% had one or more sites with bleeding, 62% had calculus and 10% had at least one probing depth greater than 3mm.[24] A continuing education program designed to increase dentists' rates of periodontal disease diagnostic notations and treatment did not result in any significant changes in patients' periodontal health indices.[25]

This latter finding is consistent with Manning and others'[26] reports on the Rand study where differences in periodontal indices were achieved only among one age group, older adolescents, who received additional periodontal services under the free plan.

Purpose of Study
To compare the need for periodontal care (in minutes) among older adults with the quantity and type of care received over two previous years.

Study Methods
The target population for our study was all persons aged 50 years and over living in private households in: the City of Toronto; the City of North York; Simcoe County; and Sudbury and District. The study sites represent a geographic cross-section of the province from southern urban to rural to northern resource-based economies and we were able to have the cooperation of the dental directors of these respective public health departments.

Subjects in the target age range were identified by means of a telephone survey based on random digit dialling. Computer generated telephone numbers were called and a randomization procedure used to select individuals from all households identified which contained one or more persons aged 50 years and over. After completing a 39-item questionnaire, subjects were invited to participate in a more detailed personal interview and clinical examination to be conducted in their own home or at a public health department dental clinic.

The clinical examination was based on methods recommended by the WHO, modified to make the data comparable to that obtained by recent surveys of adults in the U.S. The examinations were undertaken by trained dentists and dental hygienists assisted by interviewer-recorders. At the end of the interview/examination, all subjects with a visit for dental care in the last two years were asked for the names of their dental care providers and to sign a request for the dentist to release information on the care provided over those previous two years. The named dentists were then mailed the release and a two-page questionnaire.

The telephone interview was used to collect socio-demographic and basic data on oral and general health and use of dental services. The interview and examination follow-up provided data on self-reported and clinically defined indicators of oral health and treatment needs. Probing depths were measured with a pressure-sensitive probe and bleeding and calculus scores were recorded. Highest or worst CPITN scores were also recorded for each sextant where:

> 0 = healthy
> 1 = bleeding after probing
> 2 = calculus of overhanging fillings
> 3 = pockets 3.5 to 5.5 mm
> 4 = pockets 6mm and greater
> X = missing teeth in sextant

The dentists' questionnaire sought information on the pattern of care use and the date and procedure code of all services provided. "Preventive package" codes were broken into their individual procedures. Each dental procedure listed on the dentist's questionnaire was assigned its time and value unit according to the 1990 Ontario Dental Association Fee Guide.[27] All data were aggregated into specific types of service, e.g., prophylaxes, amalgams, and then to categories of services, e.g., restorative, periodontal. No downward adjustment to times or value units was made when procedures were provided at the same appointment.

Periodontal care needs were estimated using both the methods of Bader et al.[15] and Oliver et al.[16] Table 1 shows the rules we followed. The calculations required valid CPITN scores. Some dentate people had medical histories (rheumatic heart, prosthetic heart valve or joint) which precluded periodontal probing during the examination. Others refused that part of the examination. Thus, the number with estimates of periodontal care needs is less than our total dentate or service record file.

The Oliver et al.[16] published times are based on quadrants and the number of sites in each quadrant. The time estimates were adjusted downward to reflect that our data relates to sextants, but no adjustment was made for the number of sites per sextant. Thus, our estimates may be a high estimate of the Oliver et al. method.

Table 1 — Rules for Converting CPITN Scores to Treatment Needs

Worst CPITN Scores	Bader et al. 1988	Time in Minutes Following:	Oliver et al. 1989	Treatment Recommended by Oliver et al.
0	0		0	None
1	10		10	OHI
2	30		45	OHI, Scaling, Polishing
3	30		45	OHI
		For each sextant		Scaling/RP
	+3.3	Scoring 3	+20	Polishing
4	30		45	OHI
		For each sextant		Flap Surgery
	+3.3	Scoring 3	+15	Scaling/RP
				Polishing
	+20	Scoring 4	+30	

RP = root planing

Results

Response to the Surveys
To begin 33,476 telephone numbers were randomly generated and called and 3033 persons completed the telephone-administered questionnaire, for an overall response rate of 64% of eligible households. Nine hundred and seven subjects, or 30%, completed the personal interviews and clinical examinations. We received information on dental care on 518 subjects, (508 useable) which is 80.3% of those reporting a visit in the past two years.

Characteristics of Subjects
Table 2 compares the age and gender characteristics of the target population, subjects completing the telephone interview and subjects completing the personal interview and clinical examination. In terms of age, persons aged 75 years and over were under-represented among those completing all phases and

there were more women in all three groups of study subjects when compared to the target population.

**Table 2 — Age and Gender Characteristics of Target
Population and Study Subjects**

	Target* *Population* (n=436,956)	Telephone Interview *Subjects* (n=3,033)	Interview and Examination *Subjects* (n=907)	Dental Services *Subjects* (n=508)
Age:				
50-64 years	57.3	58.0	58.5	62.2
65-74 years	25.6	26.8	29.5	26.6
75+ years	17.1	15.2	12.0	11.2
Gender:				
Male	45.3	41.3	42.9	43.9
Female	54.7	58.7	57.1	55.9

* Data from 1986 census.

Table 3 compares the three groups on a number of the other sociodemographic, behavioural and health status variables obtained from the telephone survey. A comparison of subjects completing the telephone interview and subjects completing the personal interview and examination showed no statistically or clinically significant differences among the fourteen variables. This is consistent with our earlier work.[28] On the other hand, among those who were examined and interviewed, subjects for whom we obtained dental service information are different from those whom we didn't on every criterion except "born in Canada" and "oral pain in the last 4 weeks".

Prevalence of Edentulism
Of the 3033 persons completing the telephone interview, 24.1% reported that they were edentulous. Another analysis, not reported here, showed women were more likely to be edentulous than men; that the prevalence of edentulism increased with age; and rates varied from a low of 15.1% in North York to 40.6% in Sudbury. In our sample of 907 examined, 199 were edentulous, 105 either could not be probed or had no indicator teeth, e.g., root tips, etc., and 2 had no coded sex. Thus, the following 4 tables provide data based on 601 cases.

Table 4 shows the periodontal status as measured by CPITN by age and by sex. Using these scores, the oldest age group appears to have better periodontal health, given there are over 30% with highest scores of 0 or 1 and only 31% with scores of 3 or 4. Compare this to the youngest group, where only 18% have scores 0 or 1 and 47% have the two highest scores. Significant differences also occur by sex, with relatively more males scoring 4, and fewer scoring 0.

Table 3 — Sociodemographic and Other Characteristics of Study Subjects

	Telephone Interview Subjects	Interview and Examination Subjects	Clinical Services Subjects	p*
	%	%	%	
Born in Canada	60.8	64.7	66.1	ns
Employed	42.9	40.0	48.8	p<.01
Married	55.2	52.3	56.0	p<.05
Income < $20K	38.7	38.1	28.1	p<.0001
Higher education	31.9	36.7	46.8	p<.0001
Chronic medical condition	62.1	66.8	63.8	p<.05
Limitation to ADL	18.2	22.2	17.7	p<.001
Dentate	75.9	78.1	93.5	p<.0001
Chewing problem	22.0	22.8	15.9	p<.0001
Oral pain in last 4 weeks	27.1	35.3	33.7	ns
Dental health rated fair/poor	22.8	27.9	21.9	p<.0001
Perceived need for dental care	22.2	31.4	25.9	p<.0001
Dental visit in last year	62.3	65.8	91.7	p<.0001
Dental insurance coverage	47.5	46.3	49.3	p<.01

*Comparing those with and without clinical service among those examined and interviewed.

Another way of looking at CPITN data is to calculate the mean number of sextants scoring in each category. Table 5 shows these data for the 601 examined dentate subjects. Older subjects had significantly higher missing sextants and males had significantly fewer healthy sextants and more sextants scoring both 3 and 4.

Table 6 shows the estimated minutes needed to provide periodontal care according to both methods of estimation. The mean time for required periodontal care is estimated to 30.3 (Bader) or 54.6 (Oliver) minutes. The largest disparity occurs with individuals scoring CPITN = 3, where the Oliver times are more than twice the Bader times (79 minutes vs. 36 minutes). There were no significant differences by age group in these estimates.

Table 4 — Percent Distribution of Examined Dentate Subjects by Highest CPITN Scores by Age Group and by Sex

| CPITN | AGE GROUP | | | | SEX | |
Scores	49-64	64-74	75+	Female	Male	All
(n)	384	163	54	328	273	601
0	13	15	15	18	9	14
1	5	7	18	7	7	7
2	35	37	35	35	36	35
3	34	29	22	31	32	31
4	13	11	9	9	16	12
p (Kruskal-Wallis)		.044			.001	

Table 5 — Mean Number of Sextants by Highest CPITN Scores by Age Group and Sex among Dentate Examined Subjects

| CPITN | AGE GROUP | | | | SEX | |
Scores	49-64	64-74	75+	Female	Male	All
(n)	384	163	54	328	273	601
0	1.8	1.7	1.6	2.0	1.5**	1.8
1	0.4	0.3	0.6	0.4	0.4	0.4
2	1.4	1.2	1.0	1.2	1.4	1.3
3	0.7	0.6	0.5	0.6	0.8*	0.7
4	0.2	0.2	0.1	0.1	0.2*	0.2
X	1.3	1.9	2.1**	1.6	1.6	1.6
ANOVA	*p<.05		**p<.001			

Let us now turn to the record of dental services provided to the 508 older adults over the two years previous to their interview and examination. As seen in Table 7, the number of services received by individuals ranged from 1 to 37 with a mean of 10.8. The most frequent service was diagnostic (mean 3.4), of which 86% of subjects received one or more. Among those 86%, the mean was 4.0 and the maximum was 11.0. Preventive services averaged 2.2 per person and had been provided to 68% of the subjects, with a mean of 3.2 among those receiving at least one. Ninety-three percent of the group received one or more extractions with a mean of 1.2 among those receiving one. A mean of 2.9 periodontal services were provided to just over one-quarter of the 508 subjects, for an overall mean of 0.7 services per individual. These figures do not count prophylaxis as a periodontal service.

Table 6 — Estimated Mean Minutes of Periodontal Care Required by Dentate by CPITN Scores

CPITN Scores	n	Mean Minutes	
		Bader times (sd)	Oliver times (sd)
0	83	0 (0)	0 (0)
1	42	10 (0)	10 (0)
2	213	30 (0)	45 (0)
3	189	35.6 (3.4)	79.2 (20.7)
4	74	63 (18.6)	106.2 (29.7)
Total	601	30.3 (18.5)	54.6 (36.7)

Of the 5497 services, diagnostic services were the most common at 32% followed by restorative services at 25%. Preventive services made up 20% of services. Endodontic and bridge services were 2% and periodontal services were 7% of services.

Among the 508 subjects, 94% or 475 were dentate. In examining the distribution of the types of periodontal services among these 475 dentate, we need to distinguish whether prophylaxis is a periodontal service. The ODA procedure codes list prophylaxis as a preventive service and describes it as "light scaling and polishing". The periodontal procedure code 43400 is described as "periodontal scaling and root planing". Table 8 shows that, if we include prophylaxis, 84% of dentate patients received one or more periodontal services, but only 28% did so if prophylaxis is excluded. Other than prophylaxis, scaling is the next most common single procedure provided to 24% of all, followed by occlusal adjustment to 3% and flap surgery to 2%. Among those receiving one or more, a mean of 2.9 exclusively periodontal services were provided.

Table 7 — Mean Number of Services by Category
Provided to 508 Older Adults over 2 Years

	Mean (SD) (n=508)	Percent Receiving 1 or more	Mean (SD) Among Those Receiving	Maximum
Diagnostic	3.4 (2.3)	86	4.0 (2.0)	11
Preventive	2.2 (2.2)	68	3.2 (1.9)	12
Restorative	2.7 (3.2)	66	4.1 (3.1)	17
Amalgams	1.1 (1.8)	39	2.8 (2.0)	11
White fillings	1.2 (2.1)	41	2.8 (2.6)	16
Crowns	0.3 (0.8)	16	1.8 (1.1)	6
Endodontic	0.1 (0.5)	9	1.5 (0.8)	5
Periodontal	0.7 (1.9)	26	2.9 (2.7)	15
Denture	0.4 (1.0)	18	2.1 (1.5)	11
Bridge	0.1 (0.9)	4	4.2 (2.5)	11
Surgery	1.1 (0.8)	93	1.2 (0.7)	7
Total	10.8 (6.2)	100	10.8 (6.2)	37

Table 8 also shows the percent distribution of the services by category. Together, prophylaxes and scaling constitute 94% of all periodontal plus prophylactic services. Without prophylaxes, scaling represents 82% of the services. Occlusal adjustment, as a single service, is 5% of periodontal services. All other types are 3% or less.

In the 475 dentate subjects with dentists' service records, 414 had valid CPITN scores on the examination file. In Table 9 we show the CPITN scores by age and by sex. Overall, 10% had one or more sextants with at least one sextant with a score of 4. The distribution of CPITN scores was not related to age but was associated with sex. Twenty percent of females had scores of 0 compared to 10% of men. Males also showed a greater tendency to have calculus and deep pockets.

Table 9 slide shows the CPITN status at the time of examination by no visit in 2 years and increasing levels of periodontal care, from none to prophylaxis only, to periodontal care only, to both types of care. For the CPITN = 0 row, the highest proportion of healthy individuals is found in the treated groups, especially those who received prophylaxis only (19%) and periodontal care only (20%). Among those with gingivitis (CPITN = 1), the proportions increase with the increasing levels of care. The highest proportion with CPITN = 2, or calculus (46%), is found among those who visited but received no periodontal care, but the second highest (38%), is found among those who received both. If the other two categories are combined, we see that the proportion with pocketing declines with care from 49% in those with no visits to 35% or 38% receiving periodontal or both kinds of care. The Kruskal-Wallis test shows these associations are statistically significant.

Table 8 — Distribution of Periodontal Services
Received Over 2 Years 475 Dentate

(n)	Percent Receiving One or More Services (n = 475) (475 people)	Mean (Max) Services Received by Those Receiving One or More	Percent of All Periodontal Services	
			Excluding Prophylaxis (378 services)	Including Prophylaxis (1219 services)
Prophylaxis	71	2.5 (5)	-	69
Scaling	24	2.7 (12)	82	25
Occlusal Adjustment	3	1.3 (3)	5	1.6
Dressings, Desensitize, Treat Infections	3	1.9 (5)	7	2.0
Surgery with Flap	2	1.7 (3)	3	1.0
Curettage	1	1.2 (2)	2	0.6
Gingivectomy	0.4	1.0 (1)	0.5	0.1
Appliances	0.4	1 (1)	0.5	0.1
Root Planing	0.2	1 (1)	0.25	-
Sub Total Perio	28	2.9 (15)	100	-
Total (incl. Prophys)	84	3.1 (16)	-	100

As shown in Table 10, the fewest minutes of care are required by those having received periodontal services and the most are required by those who go to the dentist but received neither prophylaxes nor other periodontal services. The next highest required times are those who made no visits. While these differences are clinically and statistically significant, there still remains between 25 to 52 minutes of care needed by the most intensely treated groups.

**Table 9 — Percent Distribution of Subjects by CPITN Scores
and by Record of Previous Periodontal Treatment**

CPITN Scores	No Visit	None	Prophy	Periodontal	Both	All
		Periodontal Treatment				
(n)	(187)	(66)	(236)	(51)	(61)	(601)
0	10	4	19	20	13	14
1	5	6	7	12	12	7
2	37	46	31	33	38	36
3	32	33	34	28	21	31
4	17	11	9	8	16	12
3 plus 4	49	44	43	35	38	44

$p = .037$ Kruskal-Wallis test (corrected for ties)

**Table 10 — Estimated Mean Minutes of Periodontal Care Needed by
Record of Previous Periodontal Treatment**

	No Visit	None	Prophy	Periodontal	Both	All
		Periodontal Treatment				
(n)	(187)	(66)	(236)	(51)	(61)	(601)
Bader times	33.5	33.7	27.8	25.7	30.4	30.3*
(sd)	(18.8)	(15.9)	(18.4)	(17.6)	(19.8)	(18.5)
Oliver times	60.1	61.8	51.2	44.7	51.8	54.6**
(sd)	(36.0)	(35.6)	(37.0)	(34.3)	(37.4)	(36.6)

$*p = .004$ $**p = .012$ ANOVA

Discussion

Validity of the Data
As argued earlier, the low response rate to the telephone interview/examination stages of the study has not produced major biases in the findings on the measures we have assessed. The high response rate of dental care providers (80%) appears to be sufficient to ensure that dental services data are collected on a representative group of dental care consumers. The returned dentists' questionnaires appear to contain complete service data; in fact, some provided data from a period longer than the two years specified.

We also included service data from 38 second providers, often dental specialists but sometimes general practice dentists if the first identified provider was a denture therapist (denturist).

We acknowledge the inherent downward bias in the epidemiologic method of assessing periodontal status using CPITN. We recognize the possibility for bias in the estimates of time needed for treating the observed levels of CPITN and we present the time estimates of both Bader et al.[15] and of Oliver et al.[16] since we have no way to reconcile these.

Comparison to Other Studies
The prevalence of severe periodontal scores (CPITN = 4; pockets $\geq$ 6mm) among the 601 dentate people in our 4 communities was 13% in the younger group and 9% for those over 65. Brown, Oliver and Löe[3] found 16% in those 45-64 and 14% in those over 65. In Iowa, reported prevalence is 6.8% for those 45-64 and 2.1% for those over 55 and 65 years.[29] In the two rural counties of Iowa 15% of those over 65 had pockets greater than 6mm.[14] The NIDR 1985-86 survey found only 4% of seniors aged 65+ had pockets > 6mm.[30] Our findings fall towards the high end, but still within the range, of these estimates of United States' populations. Two other Ontario studies of independently living elderly have reported higher prevalence of severe scores in East York[5] and Ottawa.[6]

Our data show CPITN scores are worse (higher) for men compared to women and this is consistent with the findings of others.[3,14,29,30]

We have found that periodontal services are 7% of all services. Douglass and Furino[17] found that periodontal care is 4.5% of dentists' services and Grembowski et al.[18] reported that periodontal care was 2.6% of services. Thus, in this community-based sample, proportionately more periodontal care was provided compared to United States' practice-based samples.

Beck and others[29] showed that recency of last dental visit was associated with lower levels of calculus and periodontal pockets 3-6mm and 6+mm. Our data support this but show that dentate patients who have visited, but who do not receive periodontal care over two years, also have relatively poor periodontal health. They also need the most minutes of care to treat their periodontal conditions as measured by CPITN.

These findings deserve further discussion. Are others puzzled by the finding that prior periodontal care appears to have only a marginal impact on subsequent CPITN scores? For example, 82% of the "Periodontal" and "Both" treatment groups received one or more "scaling" procedures and yet their calculus scores are close to the other 3 groups who received no periodontal services. Similarly, while the estimate cannot be precise because of small numbers, 16% of the group who received the most intense level of care have a score of CPITN = 4. This is not very different than 17% of the group who made no visit and therefore received no care of any kind, and is worse than the 11% and 9% who visited but appeared to get no periodontal care that Oliver et al.[16] would deem was indicated.

Clearly, we are limited by the cross-sectional nature of our examination data (i.e., the two treated groups may have been much worse than the other three groups two years previously) and the short (two-year) nature of the service data. We hope to approach these questions with some further analysis of our data but, in reality, need longitudinal examination data to approach an answer to this.

Acknowledgements

We wish to acknowledge not only the National Health Development and Research Program of the Department of National Health and Welfare, but also our four co-investigators in the Toronto, North York, Simcoe and Sudbury Health Units and Departments, plus the many dentists and 907 subjects who participated in the clinical examination part of the study.

Endnotes

1. Advisory Committee to the Minister of Health. Dental Care for Seniors in Need. Toronto, Ontario: *Ministry of Health.* 1989.
2. Capilouto ML, Douglass CW. Trends in the prevalence and severity of periodontal diseases in the U.S.: a public health problem? *J Public Health Dent.* 1988; 48(4): 245-51.
3. Brown LJ, Oliver RC, Loe H. Periodontal diseases in the U.S. in 1981: Prevalence, severity, extent and role in tooth mortality. *J Periodont.* 1989; 60(7): 363-70.
4. Hunt AM, Lewis DW, Banting DW, Foster MK. Ontario dental health survey—1978. *J Canad Dent Assoc.* 1980; 46: 117-24.
5. Leake JL, Locker D, Price SA, Schabas RE, Chao I. Results of the socio-dental survey of people aged 50 and older living in East York. *Can J Public Health.* 1990; 81(2): 120-4.
6. Slade GD, Locker D, Leake JL, Wu ASM, Dunkley G. The oral health status and treatment needs of adults aged 65+ living independently in Ottawa-Carleton. *Can J Public Health.* 1990; 81(2): 114-9.
7. World Health Organization. Oral health surveys: basic methods. Third edition. Geneva: *World Health Organization.* 1987.
8. Douglass CW. Estimating periodontal treatment needs from epidemiologic data. *J Periodontol.* 1989; 60(7): 417-9.
9. Haffajee AD, Socransky SS, Goodson JM. Clinical parameters as predictors of destructive periodontal disease activity. *J Clin Periodontol.* 1983; 10; 257-65.
10. Loesche WJ, Syed SA, Stoll J. Trypsin-like activity in subgingival plaque: a diagnostic marker for spirochetes and periodontal disease. *J Periodontol.* 1987; 58; 266-73.
11. Ramfjord SP. Changing concepts in periodontics. *J Prosth Dent.* 1984; 52: 781-6.
12. Ramfjord S. Surgical pocket elimination still a justifiable objective. *JADA.* 1987; 114: 37-40.
13. Cutress TW, Ainamo J, Sardo-Infirri. The community periodontal index of treatment needs (CPITN) procedures for population groups and individuals. *Int Dent J.* 1987; 37: 222-33.
14. Hunt RJ. Periodontal treatment needs in an elderly population in Iowa. *Gerodontics.* 1986; 2: 24-27.
15. Bader JD, Rozier RG, McFall WT, Ramsey DL. Periodontal status and treatment needs among regular dental patients. *Int Dent J.* 1988; 38: 255-60.

16.   Oliver RC, Brown LJ, Loe H. An estimate of periodontal treatment needs in the U.S. based on epidemiologic data. *J Periodontol.* 1989; 60(7): 371-80.

17.   Douglass CW, Furino A. Balancing dental service requirements and supplies: epidemiologic and demographic evidence. *J Am Dent Assoc.* 1990: 121(Nov): 587-92.

18.   Grembowski D, Milgrom P, Fiset L. Variation in dentist service rates in a homogeneous patient population. *J Public Health Dent.* 1990; 50(4): 235-44.

19.   McFall WT, Bader JD, Rozier G, Ramsey D. Presence of periodontal data in patient records of general practitioners. *J Periodontol.* 1988; 59(7): 445-9

20.   Bailit HL, Manning W. The need and demand for periodontal services: implications for dental practice and education. *J Dent Educ.* 1988; 52(8): 458-62.

21.   Diehr P, Grembowski D. A small area simulation approach to determining excess variation in dental procedure rates. *Am J Public Health.* 1990; 80(11): 1343-8.

22.   DeFriese GH, Barker BD. The need-based demand-weighted approach to dental manpower planning (North Carolina). In: DeFriese GH, Barker BD, eds. *Assessing dental manpower requirements: alternative approaches for state and local planning.* Cambridge, Mass: Ballinger, 1982. p. 126.

23.   Sloan G. Periodontal disease in America: The unnecessary epidemic. *Oral Health.* 1985; 75(5): 65-7.

24.   McFall WT, Bader JD, Rozier RG, Ramsey D, Graves R, Sams D, Sloane B. Clinical periodontal status of regularly attending patients in general dental practices. *J Periodontol.* 1989; 60(3): 145-50.

25.   Bader JD, Rozier RG, McFall WT, Sams DH, Graves RC, Sloane BA, Ramsey D. Evaluating and influencing periodontal diagnostic and treatment behaviours in general practice. *J Am Dent Assoc.* 1990; 121(Dec): 720-4.

26.   Manning WG, Bailit HL, Benjamin B, Newhouse JP. The demand for dental care: evidence from a randomized trial in health insurance. *J Am Dent Assoc.* 1985; 110(June): 895-902.

27.   Economics of Practice Committee. ODA Suggested Fee Guide for General Practitioners. Toronto, Canada: *Ontario Dental Association.* 1990.

28.   Locker D, Slade G, Leake JL. The response rate problem in oral health surveys of older adults in Ontario. *Can J Public Health.* 1990; 81: 210-4.

29.   Beck JD, Lawson PA, Field HM, Hawkins BF. Risk factors for various levels of periodontal disease and treatment needs in Iowa. *Community Dent Oral Epidemiol*. 1984; 12: 17-22.

30.   National Institute of Dental Research. Oral health of United States adults: The national survey of oral health in U.S. employed adults and seniors: 1985-86; national findings. *National Institutes of Health*. Public Health Service, U.S. Department of Health and Human Services, 1987.

Chapter 4
Approaching Dental Care for an Individual
Patient: A Strategy Statement

Ronald L. Ettinger

Introduction

Evaluation of data from national, state and regional studies have shown that
the stereotype of the older consumer of health care being toothless or wearing
complete dentures is outdated.[1-5] Dental care for the majority of older adults
often has been an ongoing process in which an older dental practitioner
maintains a heavily restored dentition using conservative, conventional
restorative techniques. Preventive therapies usually were not a significant part
of such a treatment regimen.[6-8] If a tooth fractured, or a tooth "suddenly"
developed severe periodontal problems it was likely to be removed. If the
patient could afford it, a fixed replacement was offered, especially if the tooth
lost was near the anterior of the mouth. If not, a removable partial prosthesis
may have been used to fill the space. This process of partial loss went on until
only a few teeth were left, when a complete denture may have been
constructed. This model of dentist/patient interaction has been documented by
Marcus *et al.*[9] They examined dental treatment planning and decision making
for patients aged 60 or older and compared these decisions to those made for
similar younger patients. Their simulation study of 62 patients by 20 dentists
found that there were clear prejudices in the way dentists planned treatment
for older patients. In particular, they were more likely to extract teeth and less
likely to use fixed prostheses for older patients. Dentists were also more likely
to modify their preferred treatment plans if patients had a limited ability to pay
for care or had no insurance. Further, if patients were uncooperative or
unavailable for treatment or visited a dentist mainly for aesthetic reasons, then
dentists were more likely to modify their treatment plan by substituting less
expensive dental care. These findings of Marcus *et al.* support those of Bailit
et al.,[10] who reported that when treating minority and lower socioeconomic
groups, dentists were more likely to extract teeth rather than restore them. The
purpose of this paper is to evaluate how dentists have cared for their older
patients in the past so as to identify issues that may be significant in the future.

Treatment Planning

Traditional treatment planning is based on the application of
mechanical/technical concepts; that is, the dentist views a dentition and

proceeds to evaluate how many teeth can be technically saved or replaced without evaluating any other limiting factors except economics. This morphologically based approach has been described by Levin[11] as "the 28-tooth syndrome" and was relatively compatible with healthy patients in a fee-for-service system. Pilot[12] reviewed the literature and concluded that there was no scientific evidence available to support the advisability of routine prosthetic replacement of dental arches which have been shortened by tooth loss. Much of the information related to reduced dentition has come from cross-sectional studies. Kayser,[13] in one of few longitudinal studies, identified 118 subjects with different degrees of arch reduction and showed that there was sufficient adaptive capacity to maintain adequate oral function when at least four posterior occlusal units remained, preferably in a symmetrical position. Kayser, Witter and Spanauf,[14] in their review of the literature, concluded that epidemiological and clinical studies showed a lack of correlation between the number of occlusal units and the function or dysfunction of the stomatognathic system. However, they did suggest that persons over the age of 45 years needed at least 12 intact front teeth and 8 premolars, a total of 20 teeth. In 1990 Kayser et al.[15] suggested that there might be a relationship between needed oral function and age. They suggested that at age 20 to 50, one ought to have an optimal occlusion with 12 pairs of occluding teeth. At age 40 to 80 this functional level could decline to 10 occluding pairs of teeth, while at age 70 to 100 one might be able to function with only eight occluding pairs of teeth.

Oral Status

One of the key issues in the delivery of oral health services to an aging population is understanding what is an acceptable oral status for a particular individual. In 1982 a World Health Organization Workshop of Chief Dental Officers[16] suggested some quantifiable goals for dental care for a variety of age groups. They also recognized that oral health for older adults did not necessitate 32 teeth with an intact periodontal attachment at the level of the cemento-enamel junction. A summary of their suggestions are listed in Table 1.

Periodontal treatment needs may vary depending on the goals of dental therapy. Wennström et al.[17] have suggested that if alveolar bone height at age 75 years corresponded to at least one-third of the root length that could be considered a successful outcome of therapy. They based this assessment on a longitudinal study[18] of patients with advanced periodontitis who showed that function for a tooth could be maintained if there was one-third of the periodontal support. These articles support the work of Kayser,[13] who stated, "we should aim to preserve the strategic parts of a dentition rather than the meticulous restoration of what is damaged or missing." This progression to evaluating biological function rather than mechanical replacement in older adults still does not address the perception of need and attitude to oral health, aesthetics and function of the older adults themselves.

Table 1 — Acceptable Levels of Dental Health by Age Group

Age (Years)	Mean No. of Missing Teeth	DMF	Periodontal Status
18	1	4	0 teeth with pockets >3mm
35-44	2	6	less than 7 teeth with pockets >4.5mm
65-74	10	12	20 functional teeth

In addition, an acceptable level of oral health would include:
  A. Satisfactory prosthetic replacement for aesthetics.
  B. Freedom from pain.
  C. No unacceptable deposits on the teeth or dentures.
  D. An occlusion which is functionally and cosmetically acceptable.

Modified from WHO Workshop 1982

Clinical Decision Making

Instead of being a mechanical procedure, treatment planning should be a formal procedure that assists dentists in making relevant and rational decisions about the provision of oral health care for their patients. If a patient is relatively healthy and ambulatory, the key factors involved in providing care are related essentially to:

1. the extent of the severity of their oral diseases,
2. the patients' and/or their significant others' perception of his or her need,
3. the technical problems associated with the restoration of aesthetics and function,
4. the dentist's ability to carry out the treatment planned, and
5. most importantly, the patients' perception of the value of oral health services, which includes their ability to pay for the required care.

As long as the older individual remains healthy, few problems occur, but what happens when the long standing patient of a general practice becomes medically impaired, physically disabled or cognitively impaired? The planning of oral health care now requires the dentist to understand the wider needs of the patient, especially how they function in their environment. This includes the diagnosis and interpretation of a wide variety of factors such as medical problems, pharmacotherapy, social support systems as well as a variety of diverse sociological variables.

Historically, dentists treated the acute exacerbations of dental disease in relatively healthy children or adults. Therefore, the majority of dentists have had very little need to develop diagnostic skills that related to patients rather than to teeth. The restorative needs of these children and young adults formed the bulk of dental practice.[19] The nature of dental practice has changed and numerous studies[20-23] have shown that there has been a dramatic reduction in caries rates in children during the past 10 years. Chauncey et al.[24] have pointed out that if "coronal caries prevalence is considered in proportion to the number of teeth present, the older adults have a higher attack rate than any other age group." The recent NIDR Study of Seniors[5] showed that coronal caries was a problem for older adults and that the prevalence of root caries was three times higher in the aging population than in employed adults aged 18 to 64.

These epidemiological changes are complicated further by the knowledge that younger cohorts of elderly persons are emerging who differ significantly from their older edentulous predecessors. This new elderly group[25] has been described as being more likely to be dentate and to have higher expectations of dentistry, and less likely to accept the simple solutions of the past, such as extraction of the remaining teeth and the construction of complete dentures. Therefore, the bulk of oral health care for the functionally independent, relatively healthy, community dwelling older adult will continue to be reconstructive dental care, that is restoration of teeth and the restoration of function of the stomatognathic system with fixed and removable partial dentures.[19] The clinical techniques are usually similar to those needed for treatment of a younger person; however, typically more problems are encountered. For instance, coronal caries is often recurrent, which may mean problems with the retention of restorative materials. Recurrent caries often means that margins of interproximal restorations will need to be placed subgingivally with all the associated problems of bleeding, marginal adaptation of restorative materials, finishing and subsequent trauma to the periodontium.

Concepts related to universality of progressive periodontal disease have also changed. Recent studies[26-30] have shown that comparatively few older individuals harbour the majority of tooth sites with progressive periodontal disease. In these "susceptible individuals," even with characteristics such as bleeding on probing, probing depths of 6 mms or more and the presence of certain periopathogens, loss of attachment will increase only 20-30% during periods varying in length from one to five years.[31-35]

The decision as to what constitutes appropriate care may vary considerably for older individuals because those decisions must include a variety of age-related and age-associated psychological, social, biological, and pathological changes. Thus, for older adults, a variety of modifying factors should be identified before a treatment plan can be successfully formulated. Milgrom *et al.*,[36] evaluated 346 dentists planning periodontal treatment for seven elderly patients who wanted the best possible dental care and had no economic constraints. At the end of the exercise the investigators suggested that in general, the 346 dentists had insufficient training and/or guidelines to make informed diagnostic decisions. Specifically, the dentists had difficulty reducing the clinical data and integrating it into a meaningful diagnosis and treatment plan. Grembowski *et al.*,[37] indicated that clinical decision making in dentistry was a "social process that included the dentist, the patient, and sometimes other family members and insurers, as well." They further stated that within the process, dentists were responsive to technical and patient factors in formulating and prescribing therapy. In their sample of 156 dentists, decisions were sought between paired alternatives (e.g., root therapy versus extraction). The dentists keyed on the technical factors (e.g., age, medical history, etc.) rather than on patient considerations (e.g., patients' preference, patient's oral hygiene status, etc.) with only one-third of the dentists considering patient factors important in choosing treatment alternatives. The authors called for more research on clinical decision-making to improve an understanding of factors which influence dentists' preferences in prescribing therapy.

Treatment: Clinical Decisions

Current clinical decisions in dentistry tend to be based on qualitative, subjective estimates that a specific treatment modality will result in a net benefit to the patient. In medicine and dentistry, the traditional approach has been for the clinician to collect individual pieces of evidence and weigh and synthesize them into a subjective treatment plan, based on personal clinical experience rather than on quantitative scientific evidence.[38] There have been very few quantitative, longitudinal assessments of clinical treatment decisions in dentistry. One such assessment methodology presented by Krischer[39] evaluated alternative methods for treating velopharyngeal incompetence associated with cleft palate. The treatment methods included were the pharyngeal flap, the palatal push back, and obturation. Varying degrees of nasal resonance were used for assessing outcome. The study provided a quantitative approach to the evaluation of treatment decision alternatives. It dealt with risk and benefit associated with possible outcomes that could be applied to an individual by means of a mathematical formula.

Decision analysis has been used considerably in medicine.[40-42] In its simplest form decision making is a systematic separation of complex and confusing problems into a series of sequentially linked smaller units. Each decision is then based upon the research results and incorporates evaluation of risk and consequences. Tulloch and Antczak-Bouckoms[43] described the use of such decision analysis applied to the problem of whether or not to extract asymptomatic mandibular third molars. The outcome measure used was the number of days of standard discomfort. The difficulty in developing these assessments for aging patients relates to their multidisciplinary nature, which must take into account the patient's health status, the uncertainty of risks or benefits of treatment and lack of knowledge of the patients' preferences for the various possible outcomes. Each decision must be based upon the results of valid research and evaluate risk and consequences, however, very little information is available.

Little available research data exist on the consequences of not treating a particular condition. Early epidemiological studies suggested that gingivitis progressed with time to periodontitis and that once periodontitis was established, tooth loss was inevitable.[44] By studying untreated patients[29,31,45] with pocketing it has been shown that progression at any given site occurred infrequently and at a slow rate. Only in a small percentage of individuals did rapid progression occur. Thus, for the care of an individual, the frequency and aggressiveness of treatment will depend on determining if the patient belongs to a "high risk" group.

Berkey et al.,[46] in a ten-year longitudinal study, found that it took an average of 73 months in healthy males aged 28 to 76 years for a carious enamel lesion to penetrate into dentin. Lesions on molars in the maxillary arch progressed faster. Men with more teeth, fewer filled teeth and who were younger had a slower caries progression. Older men tended to get fewer new lesions but the progression of their lesion into dentin was more rapid. For all ages, poor oral health was associated with more lesions and a faster progression. Studies such as these are few but are important in estimating the consequences of not treating a particular dental problem. For clinicians, however, there are very few guidelines which are based on research.

In 1984[47] we developed a model to aid in decision making which we called the Rational Care Model. This model was tested when five "expert" dentists were videotaped examining an elderly person and asked to develop a treatment plan.[48] The dentists did not follow the model. This case study suggested that each dentist began the evaluation as the patient walked to the chair, then proceeded to gather data about the patient's perceived problems while also gathering data about the patient. Each dentist then carried out an oral examination of the patient and, based on the dental status and perceived need expressed by the patient, conceptualized a preferred treatment plan, which was based upon the dentist's past experience. Each dentist than proceeded to evaluate the patient in terms of the feasibility of carrying out their preferred treatment plan. When satisfied that it was feasible, the preferred treatment plan became the rational treatment plan. Thus, previous clinical experience, either good or bad, was an extremely important factor in the decision making process and the dentists relied on it very heavily.

The implications of these findings are considerable. The more limited the range of clinical experiences with geriatric patients a dentist has, the more limited and restricted will be the ability of that particular dentist to draw upon appropriate treatment strategies. Thus, it is imperative that training in geriatric dentistry, at the undergraduate and graduate level, provide a wide range of clinical experiences for dentists so that they can feel comfortable with their ability to diagnose and form treatment plans for the diversity of functional levels of the aging population.

Dental Care — Sociodemographic Factors

Successful dental care is dependent on good communication between the dentist and the patient, their family or significant others. To understand the dental needs of a patient one must understand the environment in which the patient functions; that is, one must have sociodemographic information about the patient. It is not sufficient merely to gather this information; one must understand how to interpret it. There is so much variation amongst older adults, because of their different life experiences, health experiences and expectations and their perception of need, that it is hard to generalize about any one aspect of their lives. However, certain trends based upon cohort relationships seem to allow us to make some predictions. If one evaluates only those older adults living independently in the community, it seems that the present "old-elderly," those 85 years of age and older, have the least number of natural teeth remaining and so do not seek care unless they have a perceived problem. This cohort born before 1905 is typically stoical and accepting of their deteriorating health as a part of normal aging. Individualized treatment for this cohort will be mainly prosthodontic and emergency and maintenance care of the existing dentition, as they do not readily seek or utilize dental care, because they do not value it.[4,25,48]

The next younger cohort are aged approximately between 75 to 84 years of age. Their life experiences are that they were born during and after World War I, spent their youth during the Depression and their young adulthood during World War II. On average, this cohort is better educated, and more affluent than the previous cohort. Many have retained some natural teeth, but were very susceptible to caries and periodontal disease. Based on NHIS data, in 1958,[49] 67% of this age group were edentulous. The proportion of this specific age group who are edentulous has decreased over the years to 60% in 1971 and 45% in 1983. This age group's lifestyle, socioeconomic experience, lack of exposure to fluoride, and home oral hygiene behaviours have resulted in a dentition which is at high risk for caries and periodontal disease. The few teeth that are left reflect the denture-related philosophies of their general dentists. Multiple large restoration, bulky crown margins, missing and tipped teeth and partial dentures make oral hygiene a problem for these persons with their deteriorating eyesight and loss of fine motor control. Multiple medications with potential xerostomic effect complicate treatment so that frequent recalls, innovative and personalized preventive regimens will be required to maintain the status quo and prevent further deterioration of the remaining teeth and periodontium.

The youngest cohort are the "new elderly"[25] born between 1916 and 1925 and are the most likely to be dentate. They had their youth during the Depression but were greatly influenced by their experiences in and after World War II. They are much better educated, more affluent, more politically aware and have a better understanding of the value of a natural dentition. In 1958 the 65-74 age group had an edentulous rate of 55%; by 1971 in a similar age group it had decreased to 45% and was further reduced to 34% by 1983. Declines were seen in both men and women.[49] The 1985–86 National Study reported that 27% had 20 teeth or more and 17% had 1-12 teeth. This age group reflects the restorative philosophy of their general dentists and in their adult life received some benefits from fluoridation of water supplies and the effects of modern preventive therapy. However, they have many teeth with large restorations which will require complex, coordinated skilled endodontic, periodontic and prosthodontic therapy. They are less likely to accept discomfort, poor aesthetics, difficulties in eating or speaking as an acceptable part of aging. However, what level of oral health an individual will seek and accept will depend upon their individual:

1.   socio-demographic environment,
2.   level of education,
3.   expectations of family and or significant others,
4.   level of discomfort,
5.   economic ability to pay for care,
6.   level of health or functional dependency,
7.   level of cognitive impairment,
8.   ability to reach services, e.g., geographic isolation.

Treatment Planning

The oral cavity is a psychologically significant area of the body, and when an older dentate patient seeks care it usually is to deal with a disease which develops slowly, is rarely life-threatening and where treatment may be elective. In Figure 1 a flow diagram of decision making is presented that pinpoints selected areas where decisions are required when planning treatment for an individual older patient. The first issue encountered by the dentist is that of independent decision making: Is the patient coming for treatment of their own free will or is somebody bringing them? If they are not acting independently, they may not comply with necessary recalls or home preventive behaviours.

If the patient has no dental problems, no immediate treatment is required. If they have oral problems, they may be symptomatic or asymptomatic. Many older patients are taking large enough doses of aspirin or non-steroidal anti-inflammatory agents so that acute dental infection, such as periapical infections, can occur without pain or fever.[50] The sensation of pain is extremely subjective and the dentist is dependent upon the patient's description of the site, intensity, duration and quality of the pain. It is known that the intensity and duration of pain varies greatly between individuals, depending on a variety of social, ethnic, cultural, emotional and medical factors.[51] The overriding principal is that the treatment rendered must benefit the patient and do no harm. Therefore, the primary responsibility of the dentist is to eliminate pain and control infection. In elderly patients, pain thresholds and tolerance can vary greatly, so that differential diagnoses in dentate individuals can be very difficult to make.

Once the extent of the dental problem has been determined and a possible treatment plan exists in the dentist's mind, a series of assessments need to be made. An assessment of the functional capabilities of the patient will help to determine where the treatment needs to be carried out (mobility) and how much treatment the patient can cope with. These assessments are based entirely upon experience and are judgements made by the dentist from observing the patient, talking to the patient, his or her physician and significant others. It takes a clinician time, experience and skill to sort through the body language and implied questions of these elderly persons, some of whom may still be influenced by strong cultural behaviours associated with their ethnic origins.

One of the more important decisions relates to the patient's cognitive level. Is the patient able to benefit from treatment or is their level of impairment such that they will have difficulty cooperating with the dentist? This decision is based entirely on the past experience and training of the dentist with older persons with similar problems.

It has been shown that the patient's perceived need for dental care and his/her ability to successfully tolerate dental procedures may be associated with

DECISION MAKING FOR A DENTATE PERSON

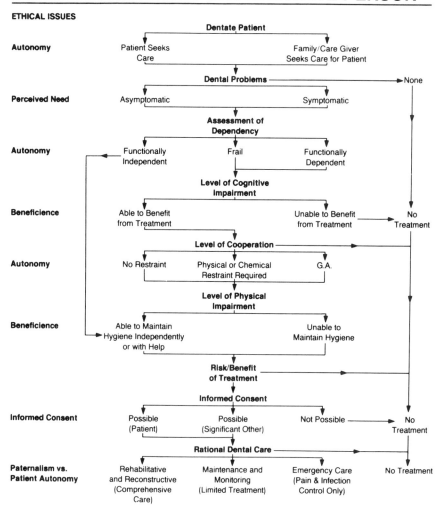

Figure 1 — A flow diagram for decision making for a dentate person.

their dental status.[52] Deteriorating oral health may signal important changes in the patient's ability to maintain adequate home care, which also may be associated with a treatable systemic condition such as depression or may be the first sign of an organic mental disorder such as Alzheimer's disease. There are no adequate research-based measures that can substitute for the dentist's experience to make these judgements. However, the primary responsibility of any dentist is to ensure the oral comfort of the patient. In many instances, this follows naturally on the elimination of pain and infection. In patients wearing dentures, it often can be achieved through the use of tissue conditioners and in dentate patients through the use of desensitizing agents on exposed root surfaces, as well as zinc oxide and eugenol cements in carious teeth. When the patient is pain free and comfortable, the dentist can evaluate the patient and the dentition with regard to the possibilities for improvement of function through reconstruction of the dentition or occlusion.

If the dentist is to go beyond the control of pain and infection, it is important to evaluate the ability of the patient to cooperate. This decision is usually based upon experience but often upon trial and error. However, if any restraint (physical or chemical) is required, informed consent to use it must come from the patient, if they are capable of giving it, or if not, from the legally responsible party, who is often a relative but who can also be a court-appointed person or institution. Before making the final assessment as to what level of treatment is possible, the ability of an individual to maintain oral hygiene needs to be assessed. Many older adults have never been taught how to adequately clean their dentition, even if they have a significant other to do it for them. Most caretakers have never been shown to care for another person's oral health. Older adults often do not understand that the primary function of toothbrushing is to reduce plaque levels in the mouth. Many have their mouth professionally cleaned infrequently. Sheiham[55] asked three questions for which there are no easy answers at this time. They are:

1. Is it essential for a person to be plaque-free?
2. Should all calculus be removed irrespective of the periodontal status?
3. Is there a need to surgically treat all deep periodontal pockets?

Interestingly, one of the few studies[53] which evaluated the relationship of frequency of oral hygiene treatment with periodontal status found confusing relationships. The analysis of time since last dental visit to periodontal status found that frequent visits were associated with less calculus and fewer pockets deeper than 6 mm, but no differences in gingival bleeding or pockets measuring 3-6 mm. In spite of these data, the value of home care still seems to be important even in the presence of calculus. Gaare *et al.*[54] in a recently published study showed that it is possible to improve gingival health, as measured by bleeding index, in persons with large amounts of calculus.

When all of these issues have been evaluated, a rational treatment plan will evolve[56] which, unfortunately, is still based upon clinical experience rather than on research. These treatment plans will be either:

1.   No treatment.
2.   Emergency care, which will include pain and infection control only.
3.   Maintenance and monitoring care, which includes management of chronic infection, restoration of carious lesion, plaque control and preventive measures.
4.   Comprehensive care, which includes surgical and prosthodontic reconstruction of function and aesthetics, including the use of implants.

Conclusions

In the final analysis, when approaching dental care for an individual older patient a number of questions still remain unanswered. These are:

1.   What is an acceptable oral status for persons with different functional levels of independence?
2.   The different cohorts of older adults have different prevalence and incidence rates for oral diseases and conditions from one another and from younger adult cohorts. How does one explain these differences?
3.   What are the risk factors involved in the oral diseases of the elderly and what are their relationships to chronological age?
4.   Are preventive procedures more difficult to apply in elderly cohorts and do they have different effects?
5.   How does one determine the amount and type of dental treatment that an individual will tolerate? What characteristics will help with prediction?

As there are no adequate answers to these questions at this time, more information is required about the following topics to try and delineate some answers.

1. The natural history of dental disease in community dwelling elderly persons, especially the frail and functionally dependent homebound elderly.
2. Treatment outcomes, especially the risks and benefits of preventive therapy, invasive therapy and no treatment.
3. Specific problems of the frail and functionally dependent elderly, especially with regard to the risks and benefits of treatment.
4. The incidence and prevalence of oral diseases in specific sub-groups of the elderly population, such as:
    a. the cognitively impaired e.g., Alzheimer's Disease and other dementias.
    b. the neurologically impaired e.g., Parkinson's Disease.
    c. the elderly diabetic patient.
    d. the chronic orofacial pain patient.

Endnotes

1. *National Center for Health Statistics.* Edentulous persons, United States - 1971. DHEW Pub., No. 74 - 1516 VHS Series 10 No. 89, Washington, D.C., Government Printing Office, June, 1974.

2. Ettinger RL, Beck JD, Jackobsen, J. Removable prosthodontic treatment needs: A survey. *J Prosthet Dent.* 1984; 51:419-27.

3. Hunt RJ, Beck JD, Lemke JH, Kohout FJ, Wallace RB. Edentulism and oral health problems among elderly rural Iowans: The Iowa 65+ rural health study. *Am J Publ Hlth.* 1985; 75:1177-81.

4. Weintraub JA, Burt BA. Oral health status in the United States: Tooth loss and edentulism. *J Dent Educ.* 1985; 49:368-74.

5. United States Department of Health and Human Services. Oral health of United States adults, National Findings. *NIH Publication.* No. 87-2868, Bethesda, Maryland, August, 1987.

6. Douglas CW, Gammon MD. Implications of oral disease trends for the treatment needs of older adults. *Gerodontics.* 1985; 1:51-8.

7. Douglas. CW. A Bright Outlook, Demographics point to a growing demand for dental care. *Dent Econ.* 1986; 76:41-55.

8. Gordon SR. Older adults: Demographics and the need for quality care. *J Prosthet Dent.* 1989; 61:737-41.

9. Marcus M, Schoen MH, Mason DT, Sue GY, Snyder YE, Hwu W. Dentist's preferences for treatment planning and their relationship to oral health status, Final Report. *University of California.* Los Angeles, 1983.

10. Bailit HL, Braun R, Maryniuk GA, Camp P. Is periodontal disease the primary cause of tooth extraction in adults? *J Am Dent Assoc.* 1987; 114:40-5.

11. Levin B. "The 28—Tooth Syndrome" - or, Should all teeth be replaced. *Dent Survey.* 1974; 50:47.

12. Pilot T. A plea against extending the shortened dental arches. *Ned Tijdschr Tandheelkd.* 1978; 85:477-80.

13. Kayser AF. Shortened dental arches and oral function. *J Oral Rahabil.* 1981; 8:457-62.

14. Kayser AF, Witter DJ, Spanauf AJ. Overtreatment with removable partial dentures in shortened dental arches. *Aust Dent J.* 1987; 32:178-82.

15. Kyser AF, Meeuwissen R, Meeuwissen JH. An occlusal concept for dentate geriatric patients. *Com Dent Oral Epidemiol.* 1990; 18:319.

16. WHO. A review of current recommendations for the organization and administration of community oral health services in northern and western Europe. *Report of a WHO Workshop.* Copenhagen, 1982.

17. Wennström JL, Papapanou PN, Grondahl K. A model for decision making regarding periodontal treatment needs. *J Clin Periodontal.* 1990; 17:217-22.

18. Lindhe J, Nyman S. Long term maintenance of patients treated for advanced periodontal disease. *J Clinic Periodontal.* 1984; 4:504-14.

19. Ettinger RL. Clinical decision making in the dental treatment of the elderly. *Gerodontology.* 1984; 3:157-65.

20. Glass RL. Secular changes in caries prevalence in two Massachusetts towns. *Caries Res.* 1981; 15:445-50.

21. Hughes JT, Rozier RG. The survey of dental health in the North Carolina population: Selected findings. In: Bawden, J.W., DeFriese, G.F., eds. *Planning for Dental Care on a State-Wide Basis: The North Carolina Dental Manpower Project.* Chapel Hill, Dental Foundation of North Carolina, 1981; 4:20-37.

22. National Institute of Dental Research. The prevalence of dental caries in United States children: The National Dental Caries Prevalence Survey 1979-1980. Hyattesville: Health and Human Services Public Health Service, 1981. *NIH Publication.* No. 82-2245.

23. Renson CE *et al.* Changing patterns of oral health and implications for oral health manpower. *Int Dent J.* (Part 1) 1985; 35:235-51.

24. Chauncey HH, Kapur KK, House JE, Rissen L. The incidence of coronal caries in normal aging male adults (Abstract). *J Dent Res.* (Special Issue A) 1978; 57:148.

25. Ettinger RL, Beck JD. The new elderly: What can the dental profession expect? *Spec Care Dent.* 1982; 2:62-9.

26. Goodson JM, Tanner ACR, Haffajee AD, Sornberger GS, Socransky SS. Patterns of progression and regression of advanced destructive periodontal disease. *J Clin Periodontol.* 1982; 9:472-81.

27. Goodson JM, Haffajee AD, Socransky SS. The relationship between attachment level loss and alveolar bone loss. *J Clin Periodontol.* 1984; 11:384-59.

28. Haffajee AD, Socransky SS, Goodson JM. Clinical parameters as predictors of destructive periodontal disease. *J Clin Periodontol.* 1983; 10:257-65.

29. Lindhe J, Haffajee AD, Socransky SS. Progression of peridontal disease in adult subjects in the absence of periodontal therapy. *J Clin Periodontol.* 1983; 10:435-42.

30. Papapanou PN, Wennström JL, Gröndahl K. A 10-year restrospective study of periodontal disease progression. *J Clin Periodontol.* 1989; 16:403-41.

31.   Haffajee AD, Socransky SS, Goodson JM. Clinical parameters as
      predictors of destructive periodontal disease. *J Clin Periodontol.* 1983;
      10:257-65.
32.   Badersten A, Nilveus R, Egelberg J. Effect of nonsurgical periodontal
      therapy VII: Bleeding, suppuration and probing depth in sites with
      probing attachment loss. *J Clin Periodontol.* 1985; 12:432-40.
33.   Lang NP, Joss A, Orsanic T, Gusberti FA, Siegrist BE. Bleeding on
      probing. A predictor for progression of periodontal disease? *J Clin
      Periodontol.* 1986; 13:590-603.
34.   Vanooteghem R, Hutchens LH, Garrett S, Kiger R, Egelberg J.
      Bleeding on probing and probing depth as indicators of the response to
      plaque control and root debridement. *J Clin Periodontol.* 1987; 14:226-30.
35.   Wennström JL, Dahlen G, Svensson J, Nyman S. Actinobacillus
      actinomycetemcomitans,   bacteroides   gingivalis   and   bacteroides
      intermedius, predictors for attachment loss. *Oral Microbiol Immunol.*
      1987; 2:158-63.
36.   Milgrom P, Kiyak HA, Conrad D, Weinstein P, Ratener P. A study of
      treatment planning: periodontal services for the elderly. *J Dent Educ.*
      1981; 45:522-8.
37.   Grembowski D, Milgrom P, Fiset L. Factors influencing dental decision
      making. *J Publ Hlth Dent.* 1988; 48:159-67.
38.   Feinstein AR. *Clinical Judgement.* Baltimore: The Williams and Wilkins
      Co. 1967.
39.   Krischer JP. A decision analytic approach to cleft palate treatment
      evaluation. *Cleft Palate J.* 1980; 17:319-25.
40.   Stason WB, Weinstein MC. Allocation of resources to manage
      hypertension. *N Eng J Med.* 1977; 296:732-9.
41.   Pauker SG, Kassirer JP. Decision analysis. *N Eng J Med.* 1987; 316:250-
      8.
42.   Baron RS, Cutrona CE, Hicklin D, Russell DW, Lubaroff DM. Social
      support and immune function among spouses of cancer patients. *J
      Personality and Soc Psy.* 1990; 99:344-52.
43.   Tulloch JFC, Antczak-Bouckoms AA. Decision analysis in the evaluation
      of clinical strategies for the management of mandibular third molars. *J
      Dent Educ.* 1987; 51:652-60.
44.   Page RC. Oral Health Status in the United States: Prevalence of
      inflammatory periodontal diseases. *J Dent Educ.* 1985; 49:354-64.
45.   Becker W, Berg L, Becker BE. Untreated periodontal disease: A
      longitudinal study. *J Periodontol.* 1983; 10:453-42.
46.   Berkey CS, Douglass CW, Valachovic RW, Chauncey HH. Longitudinal
      radiographic analysis of carious lesion progression. *Comm Dent Oral
      Epidemiol.* 1988; 16:83-90.

47.   Ettinger RL, Beck JD. Geriatric dental curriculum and the needs of the elderly. *Spec Care Dent.* 1984; 4:207-13.

48.   Ettinger RL, Beck JD, Martin WE. Clinical decision making in evaluating patients: A process study. *Spec Care Dent.* 1990; 10:78-83. 48. Burt BA. Influences for change in the dental health of populations: A historical perspective. *J Pub Hlth Dent.* 1978; 38:272-88.

49.   Ismail AJ, Burt BA, Hendershot GE, Jack S, Corbin SB. Findings from the Dental Care Supplement of the National Health Interview Survey 1983. *J Am Dent Assoc.* 1987; 114:617-21.

50.   Banting D, Oudshoorn W. The clinical management of the aging patient: Treatment concepts and procedures. *Ont Dent.* 1979; 56:19-24.

51.   Rhodes RA, Jahnigen DW, Rhodes PJ, Piepho RW. Management of dental pain in the elderly. *Gerodontics.* 1985; 1:264-73.

52.   Berkey DB. Clinical decision-making for the geriatric dental patient. *Gerodontics.* 1988; 4:321-6.

53.   Beck J, Lainson P, Field H, Hawkins B. Risk factors for various levels of periodontal disease and treatment needs in Iowa. *Comm Dent Oral Epidemiol.* 1984; 12:17-22.

54.   Gaare D, Rolla G, Aryadi FJ, Van der Ouderaa F. Improvement of gingival health by toothbrushing in individuals with large amounts of calculus. *J Clin Periodontol.* 1990; 17:38-41.

55.   Sheiham A. Dentistry for an aging population: Responsibilities and future trends. *Dent Update.* 1990; 17:70-2,4,6.

56.   Ettinger RL, Berkey DB. Chapter 5, "Treatment planning for the older adult" in Papas, A., Niessen, L., Chauncey, H., eds. *Geriatric Dentistry.* C.V. Mosby Co., St. Louis (in press).

Chapter 5
Knowledge and Attitudes Regarding Periodontal Disease Among the Elderly

H. Asuman Kiyak

A review of the limited body of literature on public knowledge regarding periodontal disease leads to three major conclusions:

(1) Public knowledge about the etiology, prevention and treatment of periodontal disease is less accurate than about caries.

(2) The population aged 65+ knows less about periodontal disease than younger age groups.

(3) Elderly from ethnic minority backgrounds know even less about the etiology, prevention, and treatment of periodontal disease than non-minority elderly.

This paper will examine the studies, both on a national and local scale, that have been conducted in the United States on this topic, and attempt to explain why older populations (especially some subgroups of elderly) are less informed than the general population. This will be followed by a description of media campaigns sponsored by dental groups and corporations to educate the population about periodontal disease, and then by recommendations on how such campaigns can be made more effective for older audiences.

Experts on the transfer of scientific knowledge and technology such as Frazier[1] report that public knowledge and opinions regarding oral health reflect the information that has been taught and reinforced by practitioners and corporate advertising. For example, even the least informed person can parrot back the message that brushing, flossing, and visiting the dentist are the best methods for preventing dental caries. In the author's own work[2,3] such knowledge was just as likely to be expressed by elderly who had not sought dental care in more than five years. Yet, this knowledge was not coupled with an awareness of *why* brushing and flossing are important in preventing caries, and how regular dental visits can assist in this process. Furthermore, this knowledge apparently has not been translated into attitudinal or behavioural change; elderly with high knowledge scores often have low scores on the perceived importance of oral health care for themselves, and do not necessarily practice the behaviours they report to be important preventive factors!

Turning to periodontal knowledge, data from the 1985 National Health Interview Survey[4] in the U.S. reveals that the public does not distinguish between preventive measures for caries from those for periodontal disease. For example, 47% of respondents in this national survey attributed great importance to fluoride in preventing gum disease and 29% stated that it was "probably important," despite the fact that there is no research evidence to support the role of fluoride in preventing periodontal disease. It is particularly puzzling why the public places such value on fluoride for periodontal conditions, since neither the dental profession nor product manufacturers have offered such a link in their public communications. As Corbin and colleagues note, "it may well be that the reinforcement of the message to brush with fluoride dentifrices has muddled distinctions in the minds of the public concerning the different processes involved in tooth decay and gum disease" (p.58). Indeed, one thesis of this paper is that the public is given messages on "how to" prevent oral conditions but none on "why" these methods are important. Thus, in slight variation from the conclusions of Corbin et al. one might argue that the message to use fluoride dentifrices has been so instilled in the public psyche that they parrot this information without understanding the function or mechanism of fluoride. Given that one objective of the Year 2000 Health Objectives for the U.S. is that at least 95% of school children and their parents should be able to identify the principal risk factors for various dental diseases and the role of fluoride in controlling these diseases, it seems that the public needs more education on "why", not just "how to" prevent dental diseases. The data from the NHIS and from Gjermo's research in Norway[5] suggest that public awareness of the causes and symptoms of gingivitis and periodontitis is woefully inadequate. For example, many people do not understand why their gums bleed.[6] Some people believe that brushing too vigorously causes bleeding gums, and, in response to this perception, may reduce their brushing frequency.[7]

The National Health Interview Survey also found that 80% of the respondents viewed avoiding sweets as important in preventing gum disease, while slightly more (88%) viewed it as valuable in caries prevention. Yet, this behaviour has not been shown in research to be important or useful in periodontal disease control, nor has it been promoted in dental health education efforts. Table 1, from Corbin et al.'s summary of the 1985 National Health Survey, also shows that the public attributes a great deal of importance to brushing and flossing in preventing tooth decay (96%) and periodontal disease (95%), consistent with the findings of Kiyak and colleagues[2,3] and with Frazier's observation of public awareness in this area.[1]

High proportions of young and old perceived the importance of regular dental visits in preventing periodontal disease (94% overall), but without data in the NHIS to assess personal dental behaviours (i.e., frequency of brushing, flossing, and professional dental visits), it is unclear how these beliefs translate into direct action by the public. A 1984 report by Brady[8] suggests that knowledge and behaviour may be unrelated in this area. In this study of new patients in a dental school clinic, 79% had undiagnosed periodontal conditions. Either these patients were not regular users of dental services, or more disturbingly, may have been patients of dentists with little training in diagnosing periodontal disease. The latter possibility is strengthened by the finding that 79% of these patients with periodontal problems reported that their previous dentist had not informed them of this. This conclusion is only tentative, since the researchers did not investigate recency or regularity of dental service utilization in this population.

Table 1 — Perceptions of Importance of Self-Care and Professional Care in Preventing Dental Diseases[*]

Response	To prevent (percent)	
	Tooth decay	Gum disease
Self-Care		
Using fluoride toothpaste or mouth rinse[1]	101	99
Definitely important	61	47
Probably important	28	29
Probably not important, definitely not important, or don't know	12	23
Regular brushing and flossing	100	100
Definitely important	88	83
Probably important	8	12
Probably not important, definitely not important, or don't know	4	5
Avoiding between-meal sweets	100	100
Definitely important	59	50
Probably important	29	30
Probably not important, definitely not important, or don't know	12	20
Professional Care		
Seeing dentist regularly	100	100
Definitely important	82	82
Probably important	13	12
Probably not important, definitely not important, or don't know	5	6

[*] Corbin et al. 1987.
[1] Totals may not add up to 100 percent due to rounding.
Source: 1985 National health Interview Survey.

Some age differences emerged in the NHIS Survey in the perceived importance of brushing and flossing for periodontal disease. For example, 88.9% of men and 91% of women over age 65 were aware of the importance of brushing and flossing, compared with 95.6% and 97.3% respectively in the 18 to 44-year-old group. This pattern was consistent across educational groups; that is, even among respondents with 16 years or more of formal education, fewer older persons perceived brushing and flossing to be important. Racial differences were also evident at all ages, especially when comparing white men over age 65 with their black peers (89.8% vs. 79.9% respectively). But no differences emerged between Hispanic and non-Hispanic elderly.

In an ongoing study by the author,[9] community dwelling elderly have been recruited to participate in an 8-week health promotion program that tests the utility of cognitive behavioural techniques with and without self-monitoring to change their oral and general health behaviours and knowledge. One of the intervention groups (n=18) was interviewed regarding their self-generated descriptions of the etiology, prevention, and treatment of caries and periodontal disease. Figure 1 illustrates the format used in these interviews.

Consistent with the findings of earlier studies reported above, elderly respondents in this sample (x age=75.4) were more informed about the cause of caries (e.g., poor oral hygiene, too many sweets) than they were about periodontal disease. More than 83% gave accurate responses regarding caries etiology; more important, 55% gave two or more accurate responses to this question. In contrast, 72% gave knowledgeable answers about the cause of periodontal disease (e.g., "plaque accumulation below the gumline", poor oral hygiene), but the remainder either did not know the cause or gave incorrect responses (e.g., malnutrition, lack of vitamin C). In contrast to their awareness about caries, none of these elderly persons had more than one explanation for periodontal disease. All respondents stated that improving oral hygiene could prevent caries, but 28% attributed responsibility for preventing periodontal disease to the dentist. For this group, personal responsibility was secondary to professional care in preventing periodontal conditions, suggesting a lower level of awareness about the importance of home care for this problem than for caries prevention. It is noteworthy that a significant number of incorrect or undocumented health behaviours were also described for periodontal disease prevention, including removal of third molars, improved nutrition, using salt water and unspecified medications, and massaging the gums. On the other hand, at least one respondent gave each of the following higher level preventive behaviours: cleaning below the gumline, using hydrogen peroxide or an antiseptic mouthwash.

This same technique of open-ended questioning has been employed by the author and colleagues in previous studies of ethnic minority groups.[10-12] The

OPEN-ENDED QUESTIONS

This section will ask your thoughts on the factors related to dental problems and dental health.

I. **In your opinion**:

A. What causes cavities?

_____

_____

B. In what ways does having cavities affect a person's life?

_____

_____

C. Can a person do anything to avoid getting cavities?

_____

_____

D. If you knew you had a cavity, what would you do about it?

_____

_____

E. Has this ever happened to you?
   If yes, what did you do about it?   Yes ☐   No ☐

_____

_____

II. **In your opinion**:

A. What causes a person to have trouble with bleeding or painful gums?

_____

_____

B. How does having gum trouble affect a person's life?

_____

_____

C. Can a person do anything to prevent gum problems?

_____

_____

D. If you began having trouble with bleeding or painful gums, what would you do?

_____

_____

E. Has this ever happened to you?
   If yes, what did you do about it?   Yes ☐   No ☐

_____

_____

Figure 1 — *A series of open-ended questions used in studies of ethnic minority attitudes about periodontal disease and caries.*

issue of cultural differences in oral health attitudes has been discussed by Mecklenburg and Martin[13] and Gift.[14] In fact, Mecklenburg and Martin suggest a sociohistorical perspective on public perceptions toward oral health, with cultures moving from an attitude of acceptance of tooth loss without replacing lost teeth, to a stage of accepting edentulousness but seeking replacement teeth, to one of restoring teeth, and finally to an expectation that destruction and loss of teeth can be prevented. Young adults in most Western cultures readily assume that they will live to an advanced old age with most of their teeth intact, albeit with some of these teeth restored. While this expectation has not yet spread widely to a preventive orientation toward periodontal disease and, as noted above, to an understanding of the etiology of periodontal destruction, younger persons who obtain regular dental care in most Western societies are developing more and more of a preventive orientation. Older persons in these cultures, as described above, are expressing more positive attitudes toward preventive dentistry, including the need for regular dental visits. But much of this has been integrated into the individual's belief system in late life, since most Western societies in the early twentieth century espoused the attitude that tooth loss and replacement with dentures was a natural process of aging.

Gift[14] summarizes five factors that contribute to a society's orientation toward periodontal health behaviours:

(1)   the extent and success of scientific knowledge transfer,
(2)   the motivation and skills of general dentists in providing periodontal care,
(3)   the availability and effectiveness of health education materials and techniques, both in the dentist's office and in the media,
(4)   the availability of environmental support systems for preventing periodontal disease,
(5)   public concern with periodontal health (e.g., in the form of community and media-initiated awareness and education campaigns).

Research findings on the etiology and course of untreated periodontal disease have slowly filtered down to the general practitioner (i.e., factor #1 above), and have led to increasing awareness on the part of practitioners in Western societies about the need to provide regular assessments of periodontal status in their patients. This appears to be more common among younger dentists and those who keep abreast of the periodontal literature. These practitioners are increasingly measuring pocket depth and attachment loss during preventive visits by patients (factor #2 above). But older patients and those with irregular dental visits are less likely to benefit from these changes in dental practice. On the other hand, research findings may not always filter down rapidly to the public if dentists do not integrate new knowledge into their patient education efforts. For example, the 1985 National Health Interview Survey[4] revealed that most U.S. adults believe that periodontal disease is the primary cause of tooth loss, even though recent research evidence contradicts that belief.

Recent promotional campaigns with public education components have been initiated and carried out most successfully by dental product manufacturers such as Colgate-Palmolive, Procter & Gamble, and Warner Lambert, which have developed some excellent patient-education materials (factor #3) for use in the dental office. Recent series of commercial TV spots also promote the value of regular dental care and attempt to teach viewers that bleeding gums are not normal. Such visual media use does serve the public in terms of easing knowledge transfer.

Unfortunately these public education efforts have not yet achieved the fifth factor described by Gift, i.e., generalized public concern with periodontal health, since the health education materials are provided through the dentist's office and therefore are available only to those who obtain regular dental care *and* whose dentists perceive a need for such education of their patients. Furthermore, such excellent educational efforts by dental product manufacturers are generally not available outside North America. In developing countries, this continues with lower awareness among dentists (often due to less emphasis in dental school on periodontal disease) and a greater focus on treating more severe caries cases than is found in North America, to reduce the likelihood of patient awareness about periodontal disease. Indeed, most of the five conditions necessary for periodontal awareness that have been described by Gift[14] are currently not being met. For these reasons, many of the developing nations today are in the second or third stages described by Mecklenburg and Martin,[13] i.e., holding on to the belief that tooth loss is natural and can be replaced by a prosthesis, *and/or* that diseased teeth should be treated. Prevention of periodontal conditions is generally not emphasized by dentists in these cultures; in fact, the public is often not even aware that periodontal disease is preventable.

The author's research with young adults from Indo-Chinese cultures[10] illustrates these differences. Although Japanese and Korean dental practices today are more likely to emphasize periodontal disease prevention, many elderly from these cultures were raised in an era when dental visits were primarily for emergency extractions and dental disease prevention was less prevalent. The author's research with elderly Korean[11] and Japanese[12] immigrants to the U.S. reflects these sociohistorical influences.

The first of these ethnic health belief studies was conducted with Indo-Chinese and Caucasian adults (x age 28.8 and 32.1 respectively) in 1980.[10] The majority of the 50 Indo-Chinese respondents were young adult immigrants from

Taiwan and China, but 20% were refugees from Vietnam and Laos. All had immigrated to the U.S. within the past three years. Both the Caucasians and Indo-Chinese represented a low-income population, as reflected in their educational levels (73% and 60% respectively with a high school education or less) and the fact that they all qualified for residence in a city-operated housing project.

Table 2 — Description of the Causes and Treatment of Periodontal Disease

	Indo-Chinese	Caucasians	X^2 Tests
Poor oral hygiene	42.5%	76.7%	8.77, p<0.003
Correct description of process	42.1%	77.5%	8.82, p<0.003
Effects oral function	48.3%	51.7%	NS
Effects aesthetics	17.9%	31.7%	NS
Correct description of treatment	12.5%	35.6%	5.62, p<0.02

Using the same open-ended approach shown in Figure 1, respondents were asked to describe the causes, process, effects, prevention and treatment of periodontal disease and other oral conditions. Indo-Chinese respondents were more likely than their Caucasian counterparts to give wrong responses (see Table 2). For example, in response to the question, "What causes bleeding or painful gums," Indo-Chinese respondents were more likely to attribute it to heredity, genetics, or luck. Only 42.5% gave poor oral hygiene as a cause, compared with 76.7% of Caucasian respondents (p<.003). Similarly, fewer Indo-Chinese knew how periodontal conditions could be treated than did Caucasians, although both groups were relatively uninformed in this area (12.5% and 35.6% respectively, p<.02). Despite being less informed, Indo-Chinese respondents had better oral health, with fewer decayed teeth (p<.001), fewer missing teeth (p<.005), fewer filled teeth (p<.005), and lower scores on the PMA index (p<.02), a measure of the severity of gingivitis[15.] Thus, in this study it appeared that the ethnic immigrant group was more likely than the U.S. natives to practice appropriate oral hygiene and nutritional habits.

In a more recent study (conducted 10 years after the one described above), a small sample of younger (ages 20-45) and elderly (aged 60 and older) Korean Americans who had immigrated to the U.S. within the past ten years were interviewed about their oral health knowledge and attitudes.[11] Oral assessments were conducted by dentists trained and calibrated in the use of several oral status indices. Neither group had a history of preventive dental visits; the younger respondents had made a preventive visit an average of 39 months previously, the older respondents 53.5 months earlier. Despite their poor history of dental care, both groups expressed equally positive attitudes about the importance of oral health and were quite knowledgeable about the etiology of caries.

However, both groups were relatively uninformed about the cause of periodontal disease, as was found in the earlier study of younger Indo-Chinese immigrants.[10] Younger Korean Americans gave the correct response (poor oral hygiene) 40% of the time, but were equally likely to attribute it to heredity or "weak gums". The remainder described the cause as poor nutrition or did not know. Nevertheless, many of the younger respondents who gave these explanations also stated that oral hygiene was the secondary cause. Elderly Korean Americans were far less informed; 39% of these respondents stated that they did not know the cause, another 39% attributed it to genetics or heredity, resulting in significant age differences in knowledge ($p < .03$). Not surprisingly only five older respondents gave a secondary explanation for the cause of bleeding and painful gums, compared with 11 of the younger respondents ($p < .05$). Table 3 presents these comparisons between young and old Korean Americans.

Consistent with these age differences in their knowledge about periodontal disease, younger Korean Americans had lower scores on a measure of gingival bleeding than did the elderly respondents, on the distal and mesial surfaces ($p < .01$), the facial ($p < .01$) and lingual surfaces ($p < .05$). These results differ somewhat from the findings of the earlier study with Indo-Chinese immigrants,[10] where gingival status was relatively good, despite their low level of knowledge. On the other hand, it is disturbing that, although ten years have passed between the two studies, similarly low levels of periodontal knowledge persist in these immigrant groups, especially among the elderly. While this group of aged immigrants was quite knowledgeable about the etiology of caries, they were uninformed about periodontal disease. This low level of knowledge contrasts even with their age peers in our ongoing study of Caucasian elderly described earlier,[9] 72% of whom could give one accurate description of the etiology of periodontal disease.

These differences in knowledge within the same age cohort may be attributed to cultural factors, as proposed by Mecklenburg and Martin.[13] The Caucasian, U.S.-born elderly grew up in an era in the U.S. when lost teeth were more likely to be replaced or when diseased teeth were repaired rather than being extracted. In contrast, the predominant mode in Asian dental practices in the early twentieth century when the Korean elderly examined in this research were in their childhood years was one of extracting diseased teeth or using herbal remedies to alleviate pain, with an acceptance of tooth loss as a natural or chance occurrence.

Table 3 — Korean-Americans' Explanation of Disease Etiology

1. "What causes cavities?"	Young *(n=20)*	Elderly (n=23)
Poor oral hygiene	65%	56.5%
Sweets	20.0	30.4
Genetics, natural process	10.0	5.0
Wrong response/D.K.	5.0	8.7
		$X^2=1.95$, NS

2. "What causes bleeding or painful gums?"

First response	*Young*	*Elderly*
Poor oral hygiene, bacteria	40%	21.7%
Genetics, weak gums	45.0	39.1
Wrong response/D.K.	15.0	39.1
		$X^2=8.93$, $p<.03$

Second response	*Young*	*Elderly*
No second response	55%	78.3%
Poor oral hygiene, bacteria	25.0	4.3
Wrong response	15.0	0
Genetics, weak gums	5.0	17.4
		$X^2=9.36$, $p<.05$

A recent study by the author and colleagues[12] among first and second generation Japanese-Americans over the age of 60 supports the conclusion above. In that study, oral health attitudes and behaviours were examined among elderly persons who had immigrated to the U.S. from Japan between 1905 and 1970 (i.e., first generation or Issei) and elderly who were themselves children of Japanese immigrants (i.e., Nisei). The second generation respondents attributed greater importance to oral health than did the first ($p<.05$), were less likely to wear dentures (28% vs. 61% respectively, $p<.01$), and gave different reasons for their last dental visit ($p<.005$). Issei were less likely than Nisei to have obtained a check-up or dental cleaning (6% vs. 63%), and much more likely to have sought restorative treatment or denture adjustment. These findings lend further support to Mecklenburg and Martin's[13] model, and extend it to cross-national comparisons. The immigrant populations examined in the author's studies were generally less aware of oral health, especially periodontal disease, than were people, young or old, raised in this country. Their oral health status reflected the effects of a dental care system that emphasized extractions and prosthetics over prevention. Finally, in all these studies by the author and others, it is apparent that public knowledge about periodontal disease lags far behind caries. Based on these findings, the following recommendations are offered:

(1) The professional associations must work with dental product manufacturers to educate the public about periodontal disease.

(2) Such education campaigns must be directed at the mass media, particularly at publications, TV and radio programs that are most watched by older adults, minorities and immigrants. Current efforts at public education via dental practices do not address those who are most at risk for periodontal disease.

(3) Such education campaigns must make a clear distinction between caries and periodontal disease, differences in their etiology and method of preventing both conditions.

(4) Greater efforts must be made by dental product manufacturers which distribute their products in developing countries to educate the public, again through the mass media, about prevention of periodontal disease as well as caries.

Endnotes

1. Frazier, J.P. Current utilization patterns of oral hygiene practices. In H. Löe and D.V. Kleinman (Eds.), *Dental Plaque Control Measures and Oral Hygiene Practices*. Oxford: IRL Press, 1986.

2. Kiyak, H.A. An explanatory model of older persons' use of dental services: Implications for health policy. *Medical Care*. 1987, 25:936-952.

3. Kiyak, H.A. and Miller, R.R. Age differences in oral health attitudes and dental service utilization. *Journal of Public Health Dentistry*. 1982, 42:29-41.

4. Corbin, S.B., Maas, W.R., Kleinman, D.V., and Backinger, C.L. 1985 NHIS Findings on public knowledge about oral diseases and preventive measures. *Public Health Reports*. 1987, 102:53-60.

5. Gjermo, P. Goals for periodontal health and acceptable levels of disease: Means and methods in community strategies. In A. Frandsen (Ed.), *Public Health Aspects of Periodontal Disease*. London: Quintessence, 1984.

6. Lange, D.E. Attitudes and behaviour with respect to oral hygiene and periodontal treatment needs in selected groups in W. Germany. In A. Frandsen (Ed.), *Op Cit*. 1984.

7. Schaub, R.M.H. Barriers to effective periodontal care. *Department of Social Sciences in Dentistry*. University of Groningen, 1984.

8. Brady, W.F. Periodontal disease awareness. *JADA*. 1984, 109:706-710.

9. Kiyak, H.A. Cognitive and behavioural methods in health promotion for the elderly. *NIDR*. Grant No. R01-DE07889, 1989-1992.

10. Kiyak, H.A. Dental beliefs, behaviours and health status among Pacific-Asians and Caucasians. *Comm Dent Oral Epidemiology*. 1981, 9:10-14.

11. Lee, J. and Kiyak, H.A. Oral disease beliefs, behaviours and health status of Korean-Americans. *Paper presented at meetings of the IADR*. Acapulco, 1991.

12. Diehnelt, D., Kiyak, H.A. and Beach, B.H. Predictors of oral health behaviours among elderly Japanese Americans. *Special Care in Dentistry*. 1990, 114-120.

13. Mecklenburg, R.E. and Martin, R.F. Oral health objectives for the elderly in the year 2000. *Gerodontics*. 1986, 2:161-165.

14. Gift, H.C. Awareness and assessment of periodontal problems among dentists and the public. *Int Dent Journal*. 1988, 38:147-153.

15. Schour, I. and Massler, M. Prevalence of gingivitis in young adults. *J. Dent Research*. 1948, 27:733.

Chapter 6
Control of Etiologic Factors of the Periodontal Diseases in Older Adults

Roy S. Feldman

The periodontal diseases have demonstrated strong associations with age and aging phenomena, although the specific role of aging in the pathogenesis of disease remains speculative.[1-6] Equally important to our understanding of clinical disease and the pathogenic mechanisms that dictate biologic change is the appreciation of the specific clinical phenomena that are etiologic to disease manifestation.[7,8] Therefore, in this discussion, attention is focused on the classical etiologic factors in dental disease, plaque and calculus, and the role they serve in concert with multiple physical, environmental and systemic factors that are implicated in the age-related pathogenesis of periodontitis. Additionally, in an era of budget constraints, fiscal imperatives and increasing need, it is recognized that management of etiologic factors in periodontitis is dependent on achievement of the greatest yield for health care dollars. This discussion also addresses the management of etiologic factors in periodontal therapy by specific dental personnel, focusing on the manpower needs and economic burdens for the aging population that are expected to increase dramatically in the next decade.[9]

Epidemiologic evidence from many studies has solidified a relationship between disease prevalence and severity and age.[10-13] Populations from opulent as well as impoverished regions throughout the world have yielded unequivocal data to support the hypothesis that disease indices increase with age, almost in an arithmetic progression.[13-15] Estimation of periodontal tissue loss is correlated with accretion of bacterial plaque, calculus and degree of oral hygiene, reliable data representing the epidemiologic scale of disease.[13,16-18] However, as current scoring techniques fail to describe disease activity,[19] we rely on longitudinal data for estimation of disease history. Longitudinal data such as those gathered in the study of normal aging by the Veterans Administration Dental Longitudinal Study also permit linking of life-style variables, hard dental data and medical information in a multidisciplinary approach to evaluate aging effects on the oral cavity.[20-21] From this approach, etiologic factors in periodontal disease may be viewed with the perspective of an epidemiologic survey but also with an eye toward the detail of a clinical trial.

Aging may be viewed as a programmed series of changes that result in unalterable deviations in anatomy and physiology.[22] Theoretically, a genetic predisposition toward selected changes may favour the development of pathology in place of normal aging.[23] The application of a genetic hypothesis to disease that arises in later life demands that we question the latency of disease to be accrued from a genetic defect. If such genetic programs are in operation in later life and are able to effect change in response patterns of the biologically active components of the dentition, in what manner would normal aging and development be more vulnerable to disease? Periodontal disease, which manifests as a cumulative assault, probably acts as a susceptible substrate for genetic disease.

Classically, the literature offers three mechanisms which are invoked to describe processes related to alterations in the aging response to pathologic stimuli: 1. chronic exposure to harmful agents, 2. alteration in immune system capability and 3. degenerative disorders.[24] Clearly, periodontitis may manifest as the result of all such working hypotheses: long term, cumulative exposure to bacterial plaque may be augmented by immune incompetence and may be viewed as a degeneration, or 'wear and tear' phenomenon in the local tissues. Therapeutically, we can describe the withdrawal of the noxious stimulus which would allow for the restoration of homeostasis in diseased tissues caused by harmful agents, and we can prescribe for the suppression of the immune or inflammatory response which would ameliorate conditions resulting from immune system alteration. It is also conceivable that progressive degeneration may be arrested by intervention at appropriate steps in biochemical pathways.[8,25] Control of disease, then, is related to control of etiology, and age-related changes in etiologic factors are critical to disease control.

The encompassing nomenclature of periodontal disease allows for the expression of the sum of the experiences that produce the clinical manifestation of loss of the supporting structures of the periodontium. The elderly experience chronic destructive periodontal disease with a clinical picture unremarkable from that seen in younger individuals.[3,19,26] Aggressive lesions typical of a rapidly progressive periodontitis may be distinguished, and over time, patterns of loss of alveolar bone and epithelial attachment seem to occur in the same clinical sites affected in other populations. Disease that remains active following therapy may be characterized as refractory periodontitis, while specific, age-related microbiologic patterns have yet to be delineated.

For the purpose of this chapter, the debate over the chronology and temporal nature of these periodontal disease manifestations is reserved for other discussions appropriate to periodontal diseases affecting other than the elderly. In doing so, we allow for comparisons to be made between different data sets based on large scale investigations of the aging process. We look at the result of periodontal disease progression over time, with the purpose of establishing common ground for discussion.

The matter of periodontal disease is ancient, as Egyptian and Arabic treatises on dental diseases catalogue accretions on the teeth and the success to be garnered from their removal.[27] This recognition of etiologic factors and their control allowed for the development of useful strategies for prophylaxis. As with all technology, the tooth brush was a marked advancement over the chewing stick, both designed for personal hygiene and directed at etiology, with some degree of sophistication in application.[27] More successful management of disease awaited greater understanding of the etiologic factors, i.e., interproximal plaque accumulation and dental floss.[28] One would expect some continued improvement in the development of local application of plaque control, especially in elderly populations, as research has been limited in this market. An application of previously available technology, the electric toothbrush, gives indication of improved efficiency in plaque removal in studies based in an elderly population,[29,30] and manually compromised elders also function better to control disease with chemotherapeutic agents delivered by subgingival irrigation, as compared to conventional oral hygiene.[31] Studies focusing on specific plaque removal systems by the elderly will continue to offer improvement in periodontal health, if for no other reason than to enhance awareness of the problem of plaque retention in aging mouths.

Biological responses of aging tissues are documented in the oral cavity, and include altered accumulation of bacterial plaque, enhanced inflammatory changes in injured tissues and decreased reparative capacity.[32-35] In a series of early clinical experiments, Holm-Pedersen *et al.* have monitored the experimental accumulation of plaque in young (20-24 years of age) and elderly (65-81 years of age) healthy mouths over four and nine days, and their results suggest that greater plaque is formed in elderly mouths.[34-35] Carbohydrate content was higher in the elderly plaque and levan hydrolase activity was lower, perhaps indicating diminished levels of streptococcal activity in the elderly healthy mouths. Other enzymatic determinations for dextran hydrolase, amylase or sucrase showed no age-related differences. These findings were interpreted by the authors to suggest that bacterial, dietary and salivary mechanisms in the elderly may account for the observed biochemical differences, and may be predictive of clinical differences.

If bacterial populations differ in the young and the elderly, then plaque turbidity and mass may favour increased calculus deposition in the elderly; high sucrose diets may impact on carbohydrate metabolism in elderly plaque samples; and diminished salivary flow may favour the bacterial and metabolic composition of the plaque sampled in the experimental design employed by Holm-Pedersen *et al.*[34] This research is salient as an example of the bridge between basic test-tube investigation and clinical observation. Although the experimental design did not allow for the estimation of dietary, salivary and microbiologic quantitation necessary to establish statistical associations with clinical phenomena, the biochemical basis outlined in these protocols may account for much observed behaviour in elderly mouths. Recent microbiologic investigations do not readily establish aging patterns in the oral microflora.[17,18]

High sucrose ingestion, as a flavour enhancer or as a self-administered sialagogue, is common in the elderly.[37] Microbiologic shifts may favour cervical carious lesions, which are strongly associated with these clinical findings, and calculus deposition may favour further gingival recession, allowing greater cervical exposure.[38-39] In this model, age-related qualitative differences in plaque composition and metabolic activity are strongly associated with the clinical development of dental and gingival disease. Therefore, although diet *per se* (i.e., high sucrose ingestion) may not be demonstrable as an etiologic factor, successful clinical therapy may require management of dietary, salivary, microbiologic and nutritional etiologies implicated in age-related disease.[40]

Etiologic factors of human periodontal diseases are most significantly plaque and calculus. Data from large scale investigations of oral changes in aging offer patterns that may help explain future practice. The Boston-based VA Dental Longitudinal Study has gathered periodontal data from consecutive examinations spaced at three-year intervals from 450 men who were healthy at the time of enrolment in the program in 1968. Three cycle information representing six years of follow-up indicated no age-related differences in plaque accumulation over the longitudinal assessment.[12,21] Additionally, site-specific identification of the dentition most frequently scored for change in plaque over time also showed no differences. Calculus deposition, however, showed interesting change with regard to the protocol of the study in that calculus decreased over all ages studied. However, as an inducement for the men to return for the three year follow-up examination, all the volunteers were provided a prophylaxis and an appraisal of dental treatment needs. In this study, therapy was not a component of the experimental protocol. Most likely as a result of the prophylaxis, calculus deposition decreased significantly overall in the first recall interval, but the oldest age group first showed an increase in calculus before a significant decrease was recorded.

In the largest epidemiologic investigation of dental health of an aging population, the National Institute of Dental Research, National Institute of Health survey of dental health of employed adults and seniors, calculus deposition seems to favour gender and regional differences.[5] Across the United States, examination of males showed evidence of greater supragingival calculus; regional differences appeared, as the east and southeastern states accounted for greater calculus than the north and western states. Coincidentally, the southern United States scored greater gingival bleeding prevalence. In both the NIDR and VA surveys, sufficiently large populations allow for statistical confidence that these observations were real, that the clinical picture is abstract and that control of disease may have to be as complex as the disease itself.

What of the clinical significance of age on periodontal tissues and what control may the clinician expect? The research of the Holm-Pedersen group in Denmark has directed important efforts towards characterization of the clinical issues in aging disease, and suggest that while the bacterial flora does not seem different between the young and the elderly in models of experimental gingivitis, withdrawing oral hygiene results in definite differences in plaque consistency.[36] Plaque from dental students was solid, compact and adherent, while plaque from healthy elderly volunteers was voluminous, soft and loose. New calculus deposition was detected in some elderly plaques over a 21-day experimental period. Gingival inflammation and crevicular exudate were accelerated in the elderly experimental group, with the healing following resumption of oral hygiene apparently similar between groups. This finding was surprising to the authors, who had expected less inflammatory response in the elderly because of diminished immunologic competence.

In a six-year study of the utility of a preventive dental health program for 375 adult Swedish dental patients, Axelsson and Lindhe have reported that when prescribed oral hygiene is successful in controlling gingivitis and loss of attachment, no age differences are perceived in the relative efficacy of the typical modalities of treatment commonly used to manage periodontal disease.[41] Moreover, in a study that approaches meta analysis as different groups of patients and experimental protocols were included in the analysis, Lindhe *et al.* showed that age *per se* seemed to have no effect on the therapeutic results following conservative scaling and surgical treatments.[42] Older individuals seemed to loose more buccal free gingival tissues post-operatively, as had been shown decades earlier by Holm-Pedersen and Löe, but both young and old benefit from therapy.[33,42]

As we accept that plaque and calculus remain the prime etiologic factors of periodontal disease in the elderly, what is the effect of these etiologies in the complex ecosystem of the aging mouth and what ancillary and supporting roles in disease initiation and maintenance do other factors play? Issues identified by the practitioner as important in the management of disease in a given patient offer a convenient window for issues that take on public health status as the population ages: i.e., xerostomia, adverse drug reactions, and environmental factors. The morbidity of xerostomia secondary to polypharmacy in the elderly is an ancillary factor in oral health in general, and is implicated in periodontal pathology;[37,43] medication abuses are commonly seen as coordination of therapy by multiple practitioners is often missing. The resultant effect on salivation is directly implicated in caries, and plaque and calculus formation is enhanced.

Cofactors in inflammation and periodontal destruction such as tobacco smoking, which may decrease vascularity in the gingival tissues as well as deplete Vitamin C blood levels and alter immunologic competence, may affect alveolar bone in periodontal disease.[1,12,44,45] Of interest is the age-related effect of cigarette smoking on alveolar bone levels: longitudinal data from older individuals show greater alveolar bone loss on radiographic survey as compared to younger cigarette smokers, and cigarette smokers had more bone loss than non-smokers and cigar/pipe smokers.[44] Presumably, cigarette smoking may enhance calculus formation and may alter plaque composition, although the effect of these factors is most likely attenuated by a compromised host response. Covariance for the accumulated calculus failed to decrease the statistical significance of the differences between younger and older smokers and non-smokers. From the results of these and other longitudinal, large scale population studies, a reasonable deduction is that cigarettes function as environmental ancillary factors in disease pathogenesis.

These issues direct attention not only to the prime etiologic factors, but also to their control in the clinical settings that characterize periodontal disease management. Towards this end of health manpower and resource planning, estimates of periodontal disease levels and treatment needs are required. Up until the mid-1980s these estimates have been based upon clinical assessment of treatment needs by an examiner's best clinical judgment or on use of several clinical indices. Treatment needs or index scores are then translated into services types. Parallel to this activity, estimates of provider time (hours) needed for each service type are made. The quantity of health services types is then multiplied by the estimates of provider time in order to calculate manpower requirements.[46-48]

In a study initiated in 1987, the Philadelphia Veterans Affairs Medical Center has investigated the costs of treating periodontitis in a population of aging U.S. veterans. Service-connected eligible veterans who had maintained at least 20 teeth were randomly assigned to one of three treatment groups:

1.   CPITN: Patients were managed by periodontist and hygienist based upon sextant-specific treatment needs identified by the Community Periodontal Index of Treatment Needs;[49]
2.   HYGIENE: patients were managed by a hygienist in consultation with general dentists and/or periodontist; and
3.   PERIO: patients were managed by a periodontist.

For the purpose of this investigation, sextants with the most severe CPITN score which are viewed as requiring complex treatment were referred to the periodontist; all others were referred to the hygienist who has the training to perform oral hygiene instructions, prophylaxis, scaling and root planing.

Throughout this study, all providers maintained the option of referral of patients to other providers for procedure-specific treatment. At the onset, providers agreed to treat and refer according to generally accepted standards of care. We report data for 117 patients, representing longitudinal results for periodontal therapy over one year. At the time of the initiation of periodontal therapy in this study, these veterans had a mean age of 57 years and ages ranged from 36 to 82 years.

We recorded services delivered by sextant and time in ten-minute units. An independent examiner scored indices of disease prior to the initiation of periodontal therapy and at annual recall in an examination that recorded recession and periodontal pocket depth for mesial, buccal, distal and lingual of each tooth and the gingival index score for buccal and lingual of each tooth. For the purposes of this investigation, gingival index scores are the sum for six sextants, and pocket depth scores are the sum of the maximum pocket depth for each sextant. CPITN sextant scores were determined independently from the results of the base-line examination for all patients regardless of group assignment. The health care providers were not notified of these scores, and were free to manage therapy as they thought best for the individual veteran. For all periodontal treatment visits, an OPSCAN encounter form was coded for treatment service, periodontist treatment time, hygienist treatment time, assistant treatment time, and operatory chair time.

In this study, two indices are used to describe periodontal disease level and one is used for treatment needs. The gingival index[50] and periodontal pocket depth provide attachment status data, and the CPITN[49] is assessed from periodontal pocket depth. Gingival indices measure the progression and regression of gingivitis according to the severity of gingival inflammation as determined by colour change of the gingiva and the degree of bleeding following probing by a progressive score (0-3) for each tooth.[50-51] Periodontal pocket depth is used to describe the numerical equivalent of tissue lost in tooth attachment. The formation of periodontal pockets is used in the CPITN as the indicator of the required level of treatment to manage destruction of periodontal ligament and resorption of alveolar bone.[52]

We chose the CPITN as an objective method of disease assessment and applied it to the delegation of health care providers. While the Community Periodontal Index of Treatment Needs was initially developed to compare global periodontal disease patterns and to calculate the type and number of dental personnel required to cope with treatment needs, since its development, the index has been used extensively to describe different populations' disease status; however, little research has been performed to determine its validity in predicting manpower and cost requirements. Additional systems of indexing health care needs in periodontal therapy have been proposed based on variations in the clinical data recorded by which treatment may be estimated;[47] however, the CPITN was most widely used at the initiation of this program. The CPITN classifies the need for therapy in each of six sextants per patient; codes are assigned to each sextant according to the "worst" finding observed in the sextant. Table 1 shows the diagnostic findings and recommended therapies for each code. This protocol was implemented for the referral of patients for sextant-specific treatment in that in the VA, hygienists are credentialed to teach oral hygiene and deliver professional cleaning, scaling and root planing, while periodontists, or dentists who are trained in periodontal therapy, are required to deliver complex therapy, such as surgery.

Table 1 — Community Periodontal Index of Treatment Needs

CPITN score	Diagnostic Features	Recommended Therapy
0	Healthy tissues	None
1	Bleeding upon probing	Oral hygiene instruction ("self-care")
2	Presence of calculus	Oral hygiene instruction prophylaxis, and scaling and root planing
3	At least one periodontal pocket which is 4-5 mm deep	Oral hygiene instruction prophylaxis, and scaling and root planing
4	At least one periodontal pocket which is 6 mm or deeper	Oral hygiene instruction, prophylaxis, scaling and root planing, and possibly complex treatment such as surgery
X	Less than two teeth present in sextant	Excluded from needs assessment

The Community Index of Periodontal Treatment Needs developed by the World Health Organization was imposed on the study of periodontal care for US Veteran patients. Sextants receiving scores of 3 or less were referred to hygienist-directed therapy and scores of 4 were referred to periodontist for management. Actual therapy provided was determined by the practitioner.

Table 2 reports the mean level of disease severity as indicated by the gingival index, periodontal pocket depth and CPITN. For this study population, mean gingival index sum for each patient was 12.66, mean pocket depth sum for the deepest pocket per patient sextant was 27.93 mm and mean CPITN Index sum was 17.60. While a slight difference surfaced in periodontal pocket depth between HYGIENE (pocket depth=25.76) and PERIO (pocket depth=28.31) groups, we found no statistically significant differences between groups for gingival index, CPITN, and number of teeth. Analysis of the clinical indices showed that the entire population required oral hygiene instruction, prophylaxis, scaling and root planing. Periodontal pocket chartings suggested that 60% of the population might be candidates for some form of complex treatment such as periodontal surgery. On average, 0.24 sextants were recorded missing and were excluded from the CPITN index. All remaining sextants, 5.76 per patient, required oral hygiene instruction and scaling, with some form of complex periodontal treatment indicated for 1.55 sextants.

Table 2 — Mean Baseline Clinical Indices for Periodontal Protocols: United States Veterans Affairs Medical Center Philadelphia, Pennsylvania

Mean Index Recorded				
Group	Mean Gingival Index (sum)	Mean Pocket Depth (sum)	CPITN (sum)	Mean Number of Teeth
CPITN n=39	12.51	28.31	17.82	23.90
HYGIENE n=40	13.44	29.67	18.33	24.93
PERIO n=38	12.00	25.76	16.60	23.68
ANOVA	0.279	0.045	0.074	0.222

Clinical data recordings for 117 patients as part of the study of periodontal therapy provided by three treatment protocols are presented according to sum for all sextants recorded. The sum of Gingival Index scores (50, 51) and the sum of maximum periodontal pocket depth are presented as the mean over all patients. The mean maximum recorded pocket depth is recorded from all teeth present and the mean CPITN score is recorded as the sum from all measured sextants. No significant differences were found between groups for Gingival Index, CPITN, number of teeth, while HYGIENE and PERIO showed a slight difference in pocket depth at baseline.

Mean baseline and one-year longitudinal periodontal pocket depth are reported for all sites in Figure 1. For each treatment group and protocol, mean pocket depth decreased over the recall interval, although no significant differences were found in the decrease across treatment groups. Mean baseline and one-year longitudinal attachment loss is calculated in Figure 2. The extent of attachment loss, established by site-specific recession and pocket depth scores, is indicated by the percentage of sites affected by loss. For all treatment groups and protocols, attachment loss increased over the recall interval, although no significant differences were found in the increase across treatment groups.

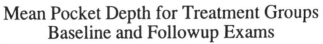

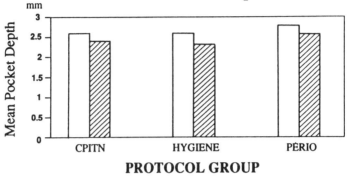

Figure 1

In Figure 1, the clinical measurements of baseline and one-year longitudinal mean periodontal pocket depth are presented for veteran patients treated for periodontal pathology according to three treatment protocols: treatment directed by Community Periodontal Index of Treatment Needs (CPITN), Hygienist-directed therapy (HYGIENE) and Periodontist-directed therapy (PERIO). Results are presented for twenty study months from 117 veteran patients as part of the study "Periodontitis in the Aging Veteran: Effect and Cost of Unmet Needs" at the Philadelphia VA Medical Center. Mean pocket depth decreased for all treatment protocols over time. No statistically significant differences were detected in the rate of pocket depth reduction.

Table 3 reports periodontal treatment time by provider for a one-year period. Periodontists spent the most time with patients assigned to PERIO (177 minutes) and the least time with patients assigned to HYGIENE (67 minutes). Hygienists spent the most time with patients who were assigned to HYGIENE (131 minutes) and the least time with patients assigned to PERIO. PERIO patients spent the most time in the operatory chair (293 minutes) as compared to patients assigned to HYGIENE (184 minutes). Patients assigned to CPITN spent less time with the periodontist (94 minutes) than PERIO Group patients but more time than HYGIENE patients. CPITN patients spent more time with the hygienist (115 minutes) than PERIO patients, but less time than HYGIENE patients. CPITN patients spent less time in the dental operatory chair than patients assigned to PERIO but more time than patients assigned to HYGIENE. Differences were statistically significant for the periodontist, assistant, operatory chair, and total provider time at the $p < 0.05$ level.

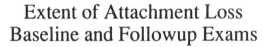

Extent of Attachment Loss
Baseline and Followup Exams

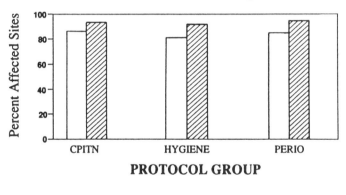

Figure 2

Figure 2 shows the baseline and one-year longitudinal attachment loss calculated from site-specific recession and periodontal pocket depth scores of 117 veterans treated by three treatment protocols. For all treatment protocols, attachment loss increased over time. No statistically significant increase was seen between treatment protocols.

Table 3 — Total Treatment Time for Periodontal Patients "Periodontitis
in the Aging Veteran: Effect and Cost of Unmet Needs"

Time (minutes)				
Group	Periodontist	Hygienist	Assistant	Operatory
CPITN n=39	94.10	114.62	140.00	222.82
HYGIENE n=38	66.58	130.79	76.58	184.21
PERIO n=40	177.44	87.44	231.54	292.56
All veterans	113.10	110.78	150.00	233.62
ANOVA p-value	0.003	0.080	<0.000	0.002

Data are presented on provider-specific treatment time for veteran patients treated in the course of the study "Periodontitis in the Aging Veteran: Effect and Cost of Unmet Needs." Time was recorded for each visit for all health care providers and for the scheduled dental operatory. Treatment was provided over twenty study months for 117 volunteer service-connected veterans on the active patient roles of the Philadelphia VA Medical Center.

The number and type of treatments recorded for each treatment protocol are presented in Figure 3. Overall, the total number of treatments did not differ between groups throughout the twenty-month window on clinical therapy. Invasive therapies, i.e., scaling and periodontal surgery, also did not differ between groups. Significant difference in the number of diagnostic services provided in the PERIO group as compared with either CPITN and HYGIENE were found by ANOVA. This study suggests that in the delivery of periodontal care to an aging population, the case manager, or the initial health care provider seen by the patient, has a profound effect on the utilization of periodontal health care resources. Additional imposition of regression coefficients for all patients show that PERIO patients (patients initially seen by the periodontist) utilized greater health care resources, provider time and operatory chair time. Assignment to HYGIENE (patients initially seen by hygienist) did not result in a significantly greater amount of resource utilization when compared with CPITN patients.[53, data not shown.]

In performing these estimates, we recognize that the following deficiencies are present: 1) when treatment needs are determined by a clinician's "best" clinical judgement, subjectivity is present, 2) indices used for the estimates have

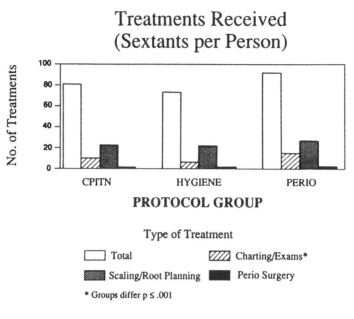

Figure 3

Figure 3 presents the number of sextants of periodontal treatment that were provided by three treatment protocols over twenty months of study. These data showing statistically significant differences in the numbers of sextants for which diagnostic services (Chartings, X-rays, etc.) were provided by periodontist, as compared to services prescribed by either hygienist or hygienist and periodontist working by CPITN patient referral. No differences were observed in the number of sextants treated overall, or in other treatment categories between protocols.

been based upon estimates of a patient's "average" periodontal disease level. When periodontal treatment is delivered, it is often dictated by the most severe level of disease, not the average level and 3) estimates of provider time assume that services can be provided by hygienist, general dental practitioner, or periodontist. How tasks are delegated between these different practitioners has significant cost implication for both public and private sectors, which are not factored into the assessment of treatment need.

Diagnostic procedures appear to account for significant expenditures of time in the provision of care by periodontists, and account for a minor component of hygienist effort. At this point, we do not know the value these diagnostic procedures will serve in the long term management of disease, nor can we identify ideal personnel to provide clinical assessments. We believe that the time allocated for a given procedure should be defined by the least expensive provider. In this regard, management of patients by protocols that identify specific procedures and assign clinical responsibilities may most efficiently treat prevailing periodontal disease in aging patients.

Why isn't chair time for HYGIENE patients higher? Perhaps the hygienist effort in patient management is projected by initial treatment of patients, regardless of disease severity. Advanced cases are forwarded to a periodontist, who assumes care for all disease. This type of referral pattern may account for decreased hygienist time. Subsequent referral patterns may be unprotected by CPITN. Furthermore, hygienists refer HYGIENE and CPITN patients according to the same criteria.

It was initially hypothesized that increase in number of teeth, gingival index, pocket depth, and CPITN would provoke increased provider time. However, step-wise regression coefficients calculated for the remaining teeth showed inverse correlation with provider time; as the number of teeth increased, the level of disease decreased. Since periodontal disease leads to tooth loss, it is not unreasonable to find that regression coefficients for teeth are inversely related to provider utilization. For CPITN patients, pocket depth was also found to be negatively correlated with hygienist time. Patients with a high level of disease are referred to the periodontist; therefore, pocket depth correlations reflect true practice patterns, in that hygienist time may be limited because periodontists assume therapy and we found positive correlation of pocket depth to periodontist time. Gingival index also correlated with provider time, although without specificity as to health care provider. Assuming that pocket depth has a higher disease specificity than gingival index and as only with significant pocket depth scores is referral made to a periodontist, it may be that specificity for gingival index scores is exceeded before pocket depth indicates referral to periodontist.

While regression models do not predict manpower utilization with great accuracy, they do help explain up to 40% of periodontal treatment time. Manpower utilization is therefore definitely not independent of the set of clinical variables suggested by our hypotheses. It appears that the optimal periodontal index for predicting manpower utilization is directly related to treatment protocol. If treatment is based upon treatment needs, *i.e.*, the CPITN index, both gingival index and periodontal pocket depth have predictive value, and periodontal pocket depth has the greater predictive value. If the hygienist is to see the patient first, the number of teeth and the periodontal pocket depth should be determined. Predictions of manpower utilization for patients who are to be seen initially by the periodontist appear to have the lowest accuracy.

In the study of periodontal disease, we lack reliable, accurate and reproducible instruments in disease diagnosis and in health services assessment.[9,19] The results of the VA study suggest that while the CPITN can be used to manage periodontal treatment in an aging population of U.S. veterans, the CPITN index is probably not very useful in predicting manpower utilization. For patients assigned to PERIO, periodontist time and to a lesser extent hygienist time can be partially explained by the level of disease. Patients with high levels of disease spend most time with the periodontist, while those with lower levels of disease spend more time with the hygienist. Certainly, these results concur with an acceptable dogma of periodontal therapy in that patients with a low or moderate level of disease may be treated by a hygienist, while those patients with a high level of disease may be best treated by a periodontist.

In addition, the VA program indicates that objective standards may be developed for the delegation of clinical responsibilities and tasks in the control of etiologic factors to specific dental personnel. A benefit of this objective assessment of responsibilities, tasks and personnel might be the establishment of therapeutic protocols for the management of disease that are easily adapted to quality assessment evaluation. Elderly populations often experience hospitalization for sundry medical problems and are frequently the population evaluated for quality assessment protocols within the hospital mechanism of peer review. The development of dentistry-specific protocols is critical in the contemporary economic and political climate, and the health services protocols we have described offer a starting point for quality assessment, in that compliance with standards of care according to an objective plan may be monitored and evaluated for specific health care providers. In the older periodontal patient, control of etiologic factors allows for successful disease management, and this population is appropriate for monitoring.

In summary, the available data describe the current hypotheses of disease pathogenesis and delineate the etiologic factors of periodontal disease without providing surprise to the clinician. In the aging population, we are clearly unified in the identification of plaque and calculus as etiologic factors, and on the age-relationship of the periodontal response to these factors. Ancillary to dental accretions, environmental factors such as cigarette smoking may influence this pattern of response. Longitudinal studies point to cumulative changes in an aging population, wherein older individuals have experienced more signs of disease as compared with younger individuals, but no direct age-related alteration in wound healing has been identified.

Management of etiologic factors in the effort to control periodontal disease appears to be achievable within multiple therapeutic protocols. Health care providers provide similar services in the delivery of periodontal care, utilizing resources with remarkable similarity. Major differences emerge in the profile of diagnostic services ordered by specialists, most likely reflecting the need to understand patterns of disease progression. Overall, success in therapy is not associated with impecunious prescription of surgical intervention. Finally, use of an objective protocol for patient referral appears to offer a reliable scheme for patient management consistent with common clinical practice. In all, the older patient is able to benefit from periodontal services and the services required to treat the older individual may be provided in an economically responsible manner. This holds excellent promise for continued control of the etiologic factors of periodontal disease in an aging population.

Acknowledgement and Dedication

This work is the result of the combined efforts of the staff of Dental Service, Philadelphia VA Medical Center.

The project "Periodontitis in the Aging Veteran: Effect and Cost of Unmet Needs" is funded by VA Health Services Research and Development #IIR-85-113. Participating in this project were Drs. Cecile A. Feldman and Alan C. Krochtengel and Mss. Anne K. Eshenaur-Spolarich and Janet A. Brunelle.

This manuscript is dedicated to the memory of Dr. Howard H. Chauncey: mentor, scholar, investigator, researcher and, at times, chief support of VA dental researchers.

Endnotes

1. Arno A, Waerhaug J, Lovdal A, Schei O. Incidence of gingivitis as related to sex, occupation, tobacco consumption, toothbrushing, and age. *Oral Surg Oral Med Oral Pathol.* 1958; 11:587-95.

2. National Center for Health Statistics. Selected dental findings in adults by age, race and sex, U.S. 1960-1962. Vital and health statistics. *Washington, D.C.: Government Printing Office.* 1965:1-13.

3. Page RC. Oral health status in the United States: prevalence of inflammatory periodontal disease. *J Dent Educ.* 1985; 49:354-67.

4. Abdellatif HM, Burt BA. An epidemiological investigation into the relative importance of age and oral hygiene status as determinants of periodontitis. *J Dent Res.* 1987; 66(1):13-18.

5. Brunelle JA, Miller-Chisholm AJ, Löe H. Oral health of United States adults: Regional findings. Bethesda, Md.: *Department of Health and Human Services, Public Health Services, National Institute of Health.* 87-2868, 1987:3-17.

6. Capilouto ML, Douglass CW. Trends in the prevalence and severity of periodontal disease in the U.S.: a public health problem? *Public Health Dent.* 1988; 48:245-51.

7. Genco RJ, Slots J. Host responses in periodontal diseases. *J Dent Res.* 1984; 63:441-51.

8. Page RC. Pathogenic mechanisms. In: Schluger S, Yuodelis R, Page RC, Johnson RH, eds. *Periodontal disease.* Philadelphia: Lea & Febiger, 1989:221-62.

9. Morhart RR, Davis ME, Weiss DG, Fitzgerald RJ, Rhyne RR. Dental health status in an aging VA population: implications for a preventive dental health care program. *HRS: Health Services Research.* 1986; 20:933-947.

10. Schei O, Waerhaug J, Lovdal A, Arno A. Alveolar bone loss as related to oral hygiene and age. *J Periodontol.* 1959; 30:7-16.

11. van de Velden U: Effect of age on the periodontium. *J Clin Periodontol.* 1984; 11:281-294.

12. Feldman RS, Alman JE, Chauncey HH. Periodontal disease indices and tobacco smoking in healthy aging men. *Gerodontics.* 1987; 1:43-46.

13. Scherp H. Current concepts in periodontal disease research: epidemiological contributions. *J Am Dent Assoc.* 1964; 68:667-75.

14. Ship JA, Wolff A. Gingival and periodontal parameters in a population of healthy adults. *Gerodontology.* 1988; 7:55-60.

15. Douglass CW, Gillings D, Sollecito W, Gammons M. The potential for increase in periodontal diseases of the aged population. *J Periodontol.* 1983; 54:721-730.

16. Socransky SS. Relationship of bacteria to the etiology of periodontal disease. *J. Dent Res.* 1970; 49:203-22.
17. Slots J. Bacterial specificity in adult periodontitis: a summary of recent work. *J Clin Periodontol.* 1986; 13:912-7.
18. Kornman KS. The role of supragingival plaque in the prevention and treatment of periodontal diseases: a review of current concepts. *J Periodont Res.* 1986; 21:Suppl:5-22.
19. Listgarten MA. Pathogenesis of periodontitis. *J Clin Periodontol.* 1986; 3:418-430.
20. Chauncey HH, Wayler AH, Feldman RS. Oral aspects of aging. *Am Fam Phys.* 1983; 28(1):131-136.
21. Feldman RS, Douglass CW, Loftus ER, Kapur KK, Chauncey, HH. Interexaminer agreement in the measurement of periodontal disease. *J Perio Res.* 1982; 17:80-89.
22. Rowe JW. Aging and disease. In: Chauncey HH, Epstein S, Rose CL, Hefferen JJ, eds. *Clinical geriatric dentistry.* Chicago: American Dental Association, 1985:6-14.
23. Rowe JW, Besdine RW. Preface. In: Rowe JW, Besdine RW, eds. *Health and disease in old age.* Boston: Little Brown and Co, 1982.
24. Andres R, Bierman E, Hazzard W. *Principles of geriatric medicine.* New York: McGraw-Hill, Inc, 1985.
25. Patters MR, Genco RJ, Reed MJ, Mashimo PA. Blastogenic response of human lymphocytes to oral bacterial antigens: Comparison of individuals with periodontal disease to normal and edentulous subjects. *Infect Immun.* 1976; 14:1213-20.
26. Pritchard JF. *The diagnosis and treatment of periodontal disease.* Philadelphia: W.B. Saunders, 1979.
27. Thomas BOA. Gerodontology. The study of changes in oral tissue associated with aging. *JADA.* 1946; 33:207-213.
28. Attstrom R, Lindhe J. Pathogenesis of plaque associated periodontal disease. In: Lindhe J, ed. *Textbook of clinical periodontology.* Copenhagen, Denmark: Munksgaard, 1983:154.
29. Robinson PJ. Periodontal therapy for the ageing mouth. In: McFarlane PB, ed. *The Aging Mouth.* London: Pergammon Press. 1986: 220-225.
30. Rams TE, Keyes PH: Treatment of periodontal patients with impaired manual dexterity—a case report. *Gerodontics.* 1987;89-93.
31. Aziz-Gandour IA, Newman HN. The effects of a simplified oral hygiene regimen plus supragingival irrigation with chlorhexidine or metronidazole on chronic inflammatory periodontal disease. *J Clin Periodontol.* 1986; 13:228-236.
32. Lindhe J, Socransky S. Nyman S, *et al.* Effect of age on healing following periodontal therapy. *J Clin Periodon.* 1985; 12:774-787.

33. Ryan EJ, Toto PD, Gargiulo AW. Aging in human attached gingival epithelium. *J Dent Res.* 1973; 53:74-76.
34. Holm-Pederson P, Löe H. Wound healing in the gingiva of young and old individuals. *Scand J Dent Res.* 1971; 79:40-53.
35. Holm-Pederson P, Agerbek N, Theilade E. Experimental gingivitis in young and elderly individuals. *J Clin Periodontol.* 1975; 2:14-24.
36. Holm-Pedersen P, Folke LEA, Gawronski TH. Composition and metabolic activity of dental plaque from healthy young and elderly individuals. *J Dent Res.* 1980; 59:771-776.
37. Epstein S. Theraputic oral health care in a geriatric private practice—a personal perspective. In: Chauncey HH, Epstein S, Rose CL, Hefferen JJ, eds. *Clinical geriatric dentistry.* Chicago: American Dental Association 1985:169-172.
38. Hand JS, Hunt RJ, Beck JP. Incidence of coronal and root caries in an older adult population. *J Public Health Dent.* 1988; 48:14-19.
39. Hand JS, Hunt RJ, Beck JD. Coronal and root caries in older Iowans: 36-month incidence. *Gerodontics.* 1988; 4:136-139.
40. Ettinger RL. Clinical decision-making in the dental treatment of the elderly. *Gerodontology.* 1984; 3:157-165.
41. Axelsson P, Lindhe J. Effect of controlled oral hygiene procedures on caries and periodontal disease in adults; Results after six years. *J Clin Periodontol.* 1981; 8:239-248.
42. Lindhe J, Westfelt E, Nyman S, *et al.* Long-term effect of surgical/non-surgical treatment of periodontal disease. *J Clin Periodontol.* 1984; 11:448-458.
43. Ship JA, Fox PC, Baum BJ. How much saliva is enough? *JADA.* 1991; 122:63-69.
44. Feldman RS, Bravacos J, Rose CL. Tobacco smoking and periodontal indices. *J Periodontol.* 1983; 54:481-487.
45. Raloff J. Smoking away vitamin C. *SN.* 1991; 358.
46. Douglass CW, Gillings M, Sollecito W, Gammon M. National trends in the prevalence and severity of the periodontal diseases. *J Am Dent Assoc.* 1983; 107:403-12.
47. Oliver RC, Brown LJ, Löe H. An estimate of periodontal treatment needs in the US based on epidemiologic data. *J Periodontol.* 1989; 60:371-380.
48. Gillings D, Solliceto W, Douglass CW. A need-based model to project national dental expenditures. *J Pub Health Dent.* 1983; 43:8-25.
49. Ainamo J, Barnes D, Beagrie G, Cutress T, Martin J, Sardo-Jufirri J. Development of the World Health Organization Community Periodontal Index of Treatment Needs. *Int Dent J.* 1983; 32:281-291.
50. Löe H, Silness J. Periodontal disease in pregnancy. I. Prevalence and

severity. *Acta Odontol Scand.* 1963; 21:533-51.
51.   Löe H, Theilade E, Jensen SB. Experimental gingivitis in man. *J Periodontol.* 1965; 36:177-87.
52.   Klavan B. *International conference on research in the biology of periodontal disease.* Chicago: American Academy of Periodontology, 1977:134-135.
53.   Feldman RS, Feldman CA, Eshenaur-Spolarich AE. CPITN-based treatment of periodontitis in American veterans. *J Periodontal Res.* 1991; in press.

Chapter 7
Clinical Experiences in Providing Periodontal Care for Older Adults in Hospital Settings

David L. Sumney

For the past fifteen years, I have been a staff periodontologist at Allegheny General Hospital in Pittsburgh, Pennsylvania. During that time we have moved our clinical facility that was on campus of the hospital, but not part of the main building, into the newly developed East Wing of Allegheny General Hospital. Allegheny is a tertiary care hospital that has a 746 bed capacity and a 96 bed capacity at its affiliated Allegheny Neuropsychiatric Institute. The new dental department was planned for many years, and on November 6, 1987, we opened this dental facility within the hospital complex to develop private care practices for patients that are a part of the hospital environment. The original facility was designed with 14 complete operatories to see patients who are visiting the hospital for related medical problems. In 1989 we evaluated 12,642 patients and in 1990 we evaluated and provided consultation for 19,118. Although designed for the development of private practices related to hospital-based patients, the service has expanded within the last several years to treat, in addition, the staff members of Allegheny General Hospital and their families.

Such a dental treatment centre within the hospital affords access to a multitude of patients who are available for treatment in this setting; yet, I feel quite frankly that the service is only developed to about thirty or forty percent capacity. Allegheny has a certified postgraduate program in Oral Maxillofacial Surgery with six residents, and it also has two full-time positions for residents in a General Practice Residency Program. I served as Director for dental clinics for approximately six years, and now I am the Director of dental treatment for medically compromised patients. I also served the hospital for approximately ten years as the Director of all periodontal services; we currently have six periodontists on our faculty who use the hospital facilities for treatment of private patients and also for hospital-based patients. It is interesting to note that the attending staff of the hospital division consists of two full-time general dentists, three full-time hygienists, two faculty endodontists, one prosthodontist, one pedodontist, four part-time general dentists, and approximately nine oral maxillofacial surgeons. The department of dentistry was recently restructured by the administration and has developed into two divisions. One division is Dental Medicine, which is in the Department of Medicine of the hospital, and the other is the Division of Oral Maxillofacial Surgery, which is a division of the Department of Surgery.

My interest in seeing patients who are visiting or confined to the hospital developed approximately seven or eight years ago, when my mother was a patient at Allegheny General Hospital. I saw the need to develop a better protocol for the development of dental needs of patients who are confined to the hospital for certain illnesses and also patients who are seen on an out-patient basis for chemotherapy and radiation therapy. I have observed, during my appointments at the University of Pittsburgh and Allegheny General Hospital, that the future of dentistry depends on care for a population which is growing older. As we reflect upon years of practice we certainly develop profiles of our patients, and I find that the older adult is becoming the basis for my current practice, both private and hospital-based. These patients are a pleasure to evaluate and treat, and I feel that they should be a vital part of all dental practices. Older people are now retaining their teeth for longer periods of time, and being a periodontist I am very much interested in seeing these patients in order to establish an excellent program of periodontal maintenance so their dentition will function for life. To organize information about such a program into functional units of treatment, I shall attempt to outline basic needs for treatment concerning the senior periodontal patient. Although this format will be extensive, it in no way implies that it is totally inclusive, and I am sure that there are other areas that could be included under this subject.

Periodontal treatment in the hospital setting can be divided into two different arenas: 1) treatment related to patients on an in-house basis and 2) treatment related to patients who are visiting the hospital as out-patients. In the United States, there has been increased emphasis on outpatient services during the last five years, and consequently this segment of the patient pool is becoming much larger.

Patients who are diagnosed as having periodontal disease while in the hospital are actually much easier for the periodontist to manage. Numerous times I am called to the specialty areas to consult with 1) patients who have been involved in extensive traumatic accidents and who will be hospitalized for two to three months for healing; 2) patients who have had severe strokes and can no longer practice any type of hygiene; 3) patients who are going to be hospitalized for chemotherapy or radiation therapy; and 4) patients who are going to undergo certain types of cardiac or transplant surgery. Because of time constraints, physician opinions, and insurance coverages, many patients undergo these procedures without such evaluation. However, in this hospital, major attempts have been made within the last five years to reach as many of these patients as possible for dental consultation. As you may know, in 1986, the American Dental Association endorsed guidelines for dental management of patients receiving chemotherapy and radiation therapy, patients with cardiovascular disease, and patients with end stage renal disease. These guidelines were endorsed, in principal, and filed for review with the counsel on hospital institutionalized dental services by the American Dental Association.

Patients whom I see in the hospital setting are usually very much interested in continuing good oral health, because they feel that the mouth is such an important organ for communication with friends and family. Thus, I find the level of cooperation in these patients extremely high. I think that there is a very direct correlation between oral hygiene and oral health. Major emphasis for reaching all hospital patients is to educate not only the patient but the team of nurses taking care of them, to accomplish good oral hygiene on a daily basis. In the case of patients who are going to be hospitalized for extended periods, due to some type of traumatic accident, they will be visited by a dental hygienist after their dental evaluation. Patients are taught the importance of oral hygiene during their hospital stay, and they will possibly receive a total dental prophylaxis at this point. Members of the attending nursing staff are very much involved in the performance of oral hygiene tasks for patients who have been traumatized to the point where they can no longer accomplish these services by themselves. Physicians who are seeing patients in the trauma unit are made very much aware that oral disease can directly affect general health and recovery for these patients, who have been debilitated through severe trauma and cannot afford to have any type of systemic infection occur. It is also important that these patients understand the importance of oral health and nutritional status. When these patients' mouths become very sore, their first reaction is to stop eating, and this may cause a slower recovery for them.

Patients who have been admitted for chemotherapy or radiation therapy are usually seen upon admission by one of the oral surgery residents or general practice residents. A complete medical history is taken by the residents and an oral examination is accomplished, noting the present level of oral health; a panelipse radiograph is taken during the initial evaluation. The physicians in charge of such patients have seen in the past that they are more susceptible to infection, oral mucositis, oral ulcerations, increased risk of haemorrhages, and impaired healing potential. Therefore, it is important to establish, in a short period of time, a high level of oral health for these patients prior to the initiation and continuation of chemotherapy or radiation therapy. It has been estimated that systemic infections are responsible for about 70% of deaths in patients receiving myelosuppressive cancer chemotherapy, and oral microorganisms have been shown to be a common source of infection in these patients.[1,2] It has been shown that removal of the source of infection in the oral cavity prior to chemotherapy and radiation therapy greatly reduces the possibility of systemic infections during suppression of the bone marrow system. Failure to remove oral sources of infection not only increases the mortality rate, but also the morbidity rate for these patients during periods of treatment. These infections, which sometimes result in an uncontrolled mucositis, complicate results of the needed therapy and also prolong hospitalization, thereby generally decreasing the quality of life for the affected patients.

The residents then confer with one of our attending staff members and a short, precise treatment plan is evolved whereby any signs of oral infections are treated or eliminated within the next twenty-four to forty-eight hours. These patients then undergo extensive instructional periods on proper oral hygiene techniques, and dental/oral prophylaxis is accomplished as a baseline during their admission testings. We desire to see these patients approximately every four to five days to improve their comfort and prognosis by avoiding delays or interruptions in chemotherapy caused by acute dental or oral disease. It is sometimes necessary to extract badly decayed teeth and those with severe periodontal involvement. However, all attempts are made to save the natural dentition in an intact status prior to cancer therapy, and many times endodontists are called in to treat odontogenic infections that were diagnosed from the radiographs. These teeth, which are basically asymptomatic, may cause an acute and life-threatening condition to develop once under myelosuppression. The nursing staff is thoroughly trained to evaluate these patients and call for additional consultations from the dental staff, if necessary. Overall, I feel that these patients do quite well, and the only shortcoming of the dental program is that all patients are not evaluated by the dental division. Dental and oral complications of cancer therapy are best avoided by treating problems likely to cause complications prior to the initiation of chemotherapy and radiation therapy. Once these patients have completed their active cancer therapy, they should be followed very closely by a dental staff member, and patients should continue their high level of oral hygiene as well as definitive treatment of dental conditions that were brought under control prior to the initiation of therapy.

Patients receiving head and neck radiation present an additional area of interest for hospital-based periodontal and dental treatment. Most oral malignancies that are treated by radiation therapy have histopathological diagnosis of squamous cell carcinoma. It is customary that these patients receive radiation in excess of 6,000 rads and, as a result, these patients are very much susceptible to radio-osteonecrosis and xerostomia. It is extremely important for the dental and medical clinicians to work together prior to the initiation of radiation treatment to reduce management difficulties and to best serve the patient's intended quality of life. Patients with malignant tumours of the oral area should have aggressive dental treatment accomplished prior to their radiotherapy, to diminish the risk associated with the extraction of teeth and also the development of infections, which are frequently more severe in irradiated bones. As a periodontist, I feel that very aggressive therapy should be initiated upon the diagnosis of these conditions; debridement procedures should be accomplished shortly following the examination so that there is a relatively minor delay in initiating cancer therapy. Major emphasis is again placed upon oral physiotherapy techniques to improve the overall periodontal health of these patients. Chlorhexidine mouthwashes are indicated. I have seen many cases where physicians or dentists outside the hospital environment are consulted and will recommend, as an end point of therapy, the chlorhexidine gluconate rinses. I feel that this is truly not an all inclusive therapy and usually does not provide the patient with a long-term, sufficient result or a completely desirable dental therapy. The use of chlorhexidine gluconate in the United States is limited to the 0.12% concentration and shows a very positive effect for short-term therapy.[3] The use of topical fluoride preparations in these patients is also extremely beneficial to diminish root surface caries involvement.[4] High levels of patient motivation must be accomplished with these patients and the practice of excellent oral hygiene on a daily basis must be employed and evaluated closely by the management team, including the nursing staff. I feel that, from the inception of treatment, such patients be recognized as co-therapists in the prevention of oral complications throughout their cancer therapy. Multiple professional dental cleanings should be accomplished for these patients in order to lessen the gingival inflammation that occurs with even the least bit of plaque accumulation. Many times these patients must be scheduled for scaling and root planing procedures in order to help control plaque accumulation and keep pocket depths to 3 mm and less. It has been documented that the presence of gingivitis in immunocompromised patients increases the risk for systemic complications.[5]

The dental and oral health care of medically compromised patients must be modified or tailored to be commensurate with the ability of the patient to tolerate certain types of dental therapy. Modification of care does not imply that such care is compromised or in any way less than accepted standards in a given clinical setting. Specifically, we realize that not all medical oncology patients are terminal and that all of these patients are able to tolerate reasonable dental care. Indeed, these patients have periods of remission and bone marrow recovery during cancer therapy. I feel that it is accepted dental practice to strive to employ reasonable technologies to decrease the probability of oral infection which could be life-threatening, especially from preexisting dental caries and periodontal diseases. This is addressed by careful attention to the assessment of caries and periodontal disease and striving to arrest such processes before an acute problem arises. It is extremely important that attending dentists with interest in this area take reasonable measures to chart dental caries, to document potential foci of infection, and probe for periodontal pockets which might subsequently lead to periodontal abscess formation. To enhance their diagnosis, appropriate screening panoramic radiographs must be taken to rule out diseases which could be catastrophic in a patient receiving a cytotoxic medication. Such oral treatments which have predictive value prior to or during cancer therapy include treatment of exposed impacted teeth, cysts, chronic dentoalveolar infections or apical granulomas, deep periodontal infrabony pockets, advanced caries, endodontically treated teeth, chronically infected paranasal sinuses (maxillary), and possible neoplastic processes involving the jaws.

Patients who are diagnosed for certain cardiovascular diseases requiring surgical correction, such as valve replacements and coronary artery bypass procedures, are compromised patients and should be evaluated by a dental team. In our hospital setting, numerous referrals from cardiovascular surgeons are made in order to determine the dental health status of these patients prior to the initiation of cardiac surgery. Unfortunately, a number of patients who develop complications to valve replacements that were not screened prior to the initiation of cardiovascular surgery are also seen postsurgically. The communication between dentists and physicians responsible for patient care is essential in these compromised patients. It is extremely important to assure that appropriate antibiotic prophylaxis be followed for all patients to reduce the risk of post-treatment infectious endocarditis, as recommended by the American Heart Association. It is also important to establish a state of oral health that will decrease the risk of infection and subsequent bacteraemia. Periodontal disease is usually seen in this group of patients, who are often between the fourth and seventh decades of life. The timing of dental treatment and sequencing of dental and medical care are extremely important for patients awaiting valve replacement or six months after myocardial infarction or bypass surgery. It is sometimes necessary for adjustment of medications such as those utilized in anticoagulation therapy; thus close communication between the physician and periodontist is extremely important. Protocol would dictate that patients receive appropriate clinical and radiographic dental evaluations to assess their dental needs at the time that the cardiovascular problem is diagnosed. Dental treatment recommendations should be designed according to acceptable dental practice with specific consideration for the patient's cardiovascular status risk factors, restrictions, limitations, and prognosis. Patients who are in need of coronary bypass surgery should have dental treatment delayed approximately three to six months to assure that the bypass surgery has improved the myocardial reserve, and necessary periodontal treatment should be accomplished utilizing techniques that are objective and that produce the desired results in a short period of time. I very much recommend that treatment of these patients be accomplished in one appointment utilizing intravenous conscious sedation. In most instances, following dental consultation, patients in need of heart transplants or valve replacements are treated in an operating room setting utilizing surgical techniques that will eliminate inflammation in tissues with periodontitis. Both active and potential sources of infection are eliminated during this appointment, and the patient is immediately returned to his/her room for extensive follow-up care relative to adequate oral hygiene procedures. These patients are covered pre-operatively and post-operatively by antibiotic therapy. Those who are on immunosuppressive agents following heart transplants are the most challenging for long-term establishment of periodontal health. Use of immunosuppressive medications many times results in gingival overgrowth that is difficult to manage unless the patient is extremely well educated in daily plaque control and also personally designed gingival stimulation techniques.

Another group of patients whom we see in the hospital setting for moderate periods of time are patients with end stage renal diseases. These individuals are usually very ill. They have a variety of metabolic abnormalities including impaired excretory capacity, fluid and electrolyte imbalance, moderate to severe hypertension, anaemia, bleeding problems, and altered drug metabolisms. These patients are usually on well-designed dialysis programs and are regulated prior to their discharge. Because these patients are very susceptible to infections, it is important that a dental evaluation be made during their hospital visit.[6] Adequate pretreatment dental evaluations and dental treatment with proper consideration for the patient's renal status and related problems should prevent significant complications.[7] Many of these patients eventually have kidney transplants and again are susceptible to gingival hyperplasia secondary to cyclosporin therapy. It is also important to realize that these patients usually have increased incidence of hypertension; thus drug doses are very much affected because renal excretion is compromised. Prior to kidney transplantation, dental treatment is extremely important in older to stabilize existing deteriorating conditions and also to educate the patient in the proper oral hygiene techniques specifically designed for their needs. The extensive dental examination of these patients detects changes in the bone profile consistent with renal osteodystrophy, eremic mucosal lesions, and enamel hypoplasia. Prior to renal transplantation, periodontal and perioicoronal sources of bacteraemia should be identified and eliminated, if possible.[8] Because these patients are usually in-house for a minimum of five to seven days prior to kidney transplant procedures, necessary dental treatment can be initiated and completed utilizing comprehensive treatment techniques. Like cardiovascular patients, renal disease patients are usually treated for quick elimination of periodontal inflammation by conservative surgical techniques consisting of modified Widman flaps and thorough root planing and scaling. This can usually be accomplished in approximately two hours under intravenous conscious sedation; such patients have a quick and optimistic recovery period. During the period of additional medical testing, these patients are usually visited two to three times a week in order to emphasize plaque control measures which are necessary for them to complete on a daily basis and also to evaluate the oral mucosa for possible ulcerations.

Hospital patients are usually quite cooperative, and the advantage of seeing them in a hospital setting is that it really does help to take their mind off their more serious medical problems. They are usually delighted that we show such a keen interest in their overall health as well as their dental health. The advantage of seeing these patients is that it opens up a great line of communication for both them and their families, and many times referral of their friends and families for periodontal diagnosis and treatment are made by patients once they leave the hospital setting. I feel that it is necessary for all members of the dental team to display an attitude of total compassion for patients who are hospitalized for these very serious medical conditions. The dental aspect of their treatment is important, but most of them have focused upon prolonging their lives through complicated and expensive medical surgical treatments. It has been my experience that upon discharge from the hospital setting these patients continue to visit me for dental evaluations and also for periodontal maintenance for extended periods of time. They understand the importance of good oral health and are more than happy to cooperate in long-term periodontal maintenance programs.[9] These patients are taught that poor oral hygiene is considered an important contributing factor to recurrent oral diseases, and most of them have had some level of sophisticated dentistry accomplished in the past and would like to continue to retain their natural, functioning dentition.

It is also important to note that because of advancements in implant dentistry, a number of patients whom I see have already undergone dental implant procedures of various kinds prior to their development of medical problems. It is extremely important to understand that implant sites are areas of potential infection, and major emphasis should be placed on teaching patients that these implant areas must be maintained to the same level of periodontal care as areas of natural dentition. It has been my experience that most patients, both in the hospital setting and in private practice, think that dental implants are lifetime dental prostheses, and they have not been taught that implants are susceptible to "periodontal" disease just as their natural teeth had been prior to their extraction. In examining patients in a hospital setting, it is important to pay attention to not only the periodontium and teeth, but also to the appearance of the gingival mucosa, the tongue, the roof and floor of the mouth, and the lips. In evaluating these patients, an ill-fitting prosthesis is often found, and although the patient may have mentioned it to their dentist, it has been overlooked. Once these patients are feeling well, we appoint them to the main dental centre for a series of visits to make adjustments or reline their prosthetic appliances. It is also important at all times to pay attention to the saliva during the early examination of these patients. Many of them, prior to their admission, have taken antihistamines, antihypertensives, antidepressants, diuretics, cardiac medications, and narcotic analgesics. This can cause a shift in the type and quantity of saliva that is being produced and these patients often have altered sensations in their mouth, which should be addressed. Some patients have a gingival recession pattern that would be conducive to the development of root surface caries after gingival shrinkage and elimination of gingival inflammation. Special attempts should be made to advise these patients about diet control, use of fluoridated toothpaste, and also about how to manage the sensitivity of the root surfaces many of them experience following periodontal treatment.

The other major group of patients which is seen as out-patients in the dental facility consists of older adults. Many of these patients should have been seen as patients in the hospital. In any event, many older patients are referred for routine periodontal care by our and other hospitals in the greater Pittsburgh area, as well as by area clinicians. I feel that the medical profession is sometimes filled with biases and misconceptions about older adults. With the increasing life expectancy in economically developed countries, we are very much becoming an international nation of older people. The state in which I practice, Pennsylvania, has the third highest proportion of people over sixty-five in the United States. It is estimated that by the year 2000 there may be as many as 32 million elderly Americans comprising approximately 15% of the total population, and half of these people will be over the age of seventy five.[10] The population that I see as periodontal patients, both in my private practice and my practice at the hospital, are usually in very good to excellent physical condition and have astute mental responses. Many of them have had sophisticated dental procedures such as implants placed several years ago. This group of patients has the time to read a great deal and is usually very current in their thoughts and knowledge about medicine and dentistry. Again, as a periodontist, I do see a certain segment of the population that has usually had fairly good dental care in the past and continues to be interested in saving their teeth. As an overall evaluation, I think that older citizens are now taking very good care of themselves, both medically and dentally.

It is important that clinicians understand the difference between normal aging and pathological changes. Through efforts in continuing education, I feel that dental staffs are now better trained to understand the periodontal and dental needs of older adults and are in a position to provide appropriate care for these individuals. In the out-patient hospital setting, it is extremely important that an accurate medical and dental history be taken on each patient. This usually requires approximately twenty to twenty-five minutes of time by myself and my staff in order to evaluate the patient from a medical and dental point of view. People older than age sixty-five account for use of approximately 25 to 30% of all medical services, and account for 25% to 30% of all U.S. drug expenditures. Approximately 85% of the ambulatory elderly are taking medications of some type on a daily basis.[12] It has not been my experience in treating elderly patients that the healing responses in older individuals is impaired in any way. In fact, I find that these patients, because of their high level of participation in their treatment, have excellent surgical responses, and more importantly are probably the very best group of people for periodontal maintenance. Many times I have obtained excellent surgical and clinical results in thirty- to forty-year-old individuals to find that they eventually drop out of the maintenance program that has been established for them, because they perceive no problems. I do not see this trend in older individuals. As long as they are able to get around and make their visits, they are more than happy to come in for their checkups and periodic periodontal maintenance.

By far, the most prevalent periodontal problem that I see in elderly adults is gingival recession. One of the proposed reasons for recession is normal biological loss of bone support for the overlying soft tissues.[13] In other words, the longer one lives the more gingival recession might be experienced. There are other reasons cited for gingival recession with time, such as the wearing of the gingival tissue through normal mastication and also through faulty brushing techniques. Gingival recession is a detrimental process to the total oral health of the patient due mostly to the risk for development of root surface caries on exposed cemental surfaces. I find that patients with gingival recession many times refer themselves because they notice that this tends to be a progressive situation, and they get concerned from both an aesthetic and functional point of view. Patients with gingival recession should be treated to stabilize this condition. Recession should be treated in this group of patients in a similar fashion to recession in younger age groups. This may involve surgical procedures to arrest the condition and prevent apical migration of the dentogingival attachment. When necessary, I treat these patients with surgical procedures such as periodontal grafts, mucogingival procedures, and routine scaling and root planing in order to prevent further recession from developing. In this group of patients, pocket depths greater than 6 mm are seldom detected, and tissue response to surgical procedures is quite good.

Again, in suggesting surgical treatment to this group of older adults, it is extremely important to emphasize that an accurate medical history be obtained and physicians be consulted about the medications that their patients are taking. Lindhe et al.[14] demonstrated that older and younger patients with moderate and severe periodontitis showed equal abilities to heal. They indicated that the elderly patient can be treated successfully with periodontal therapy, and the dentition can be maintained for many years. Most clinicians agree that an elderly patient with moderate bone loss patterns has a better periodontal prognosis than a young patient with the same amount of bone loss and gingival inflammation. Elderly patients seen in the hospital setting usually have varying degrees of periodontal involvement. Some of these patients are treated with major emphasis on oral physiotherapy and root planing and then periodontal maintenance. However, most patients fall into the moderate to moderately advanced periodontitis classifications for which treatment requires increased emphasis on home care instructions, an initial debridement phase, and a phase for specified surgical corrections in certain areas, and finally a vigorous periodontal maintenance program.

We have developed a system of treatment by which medically compromised patients in need of periodontal surgical treatment are treated for surgical needs in one appointment utilizing intravenous conscious sedation. Approximately ten patients per week are treated following this protocol. There are many advantages in that patients are extremely well controlled and managed medically because all of our sedations are administered by medical or dental anesthesiologists. Treatment is expedited and the number of visits that the patient has to make minimized. These patients most often have an uneventful healing period. They are sedated to the point where they are extremely relaxed during their therapy and they have very low levels of anxiety. Most of them also receive a steroid intravenously in order to minimize postoperative swelling reactions. Periodontal dressings are applied to the treated areas and left in place for approximately five to seven days and then removed. The patients are seen approximately three more times prior to the initiation of the maintenance phase of their periodontal treatment.

Very few patients seen in the elderly age group have advanced periodontal disease. I feel that the reason for this is probably that, through the years, periodontally involved teeth were extracted and many of these patients end up wearing partial or even full dentures. However, patients who do have remaining teeth are quite interested in treatment. Subsequent tooth loss has not been a problem among patients in this age group whom I have treated. As stated previously, these patients are placed in a vigorous periodontal maintenance program. They are quite dependable at keeping appointments for the review of plaque control, topical fluoride applications, and isolated areas of root planing and scaling, as well as routine dental cleanings.

Treatment planning for older periodontal patients is quite exciting and usually involves a number of different restorative approaches to repair the badly worn teeth. In the hospital setting, I work with three excellent general dentists and an attending prosthodontist. We have in a number of cases in the last three years recommended dental implants of varying types. I find that many of the patients who have presented for periodontal consultation have not seen dentists for many years and are wearing dental prostheses that are ill fitting and, in some instances, actually broken and carried in hand to the appointment. I think that some older people feel that dentists are not really interested in treating them, and after age sixty-five or seventy they drop out of routine dental practices. For some reason, these practices neither pursue nor attract them back into active treatment.

In summary, I am delighted to have a large segment of my patient population as older periodontal patients. We have developed an extensive rapport with physicians in the area, who continue to refer patients to us because of the lines of communication that we have established concerning the medical profiles of patients whom we have seen. This is one area of referral that continues to develop. By treating older periodontal patients and making them feel very comfortable and satisfied with our proposed treatments, we have been able to generate numerous referrals for periodontal consultation among their children and even grandchildren. Developing this type of family practice is one of the many rewards in treating this cohort of patients. Overall, I view the senior periodontal patient as a patient who is extremely cooperative, who usually follows through with recommended treatment, and who often has the financial means and integrity to pay the associated fees for services.

Endnotes

1.   McElroy TH. Infection in the patient receiving chemotherapy: oral considerations. *JADA*. 1984; 109:454.

2.   Peterson DE, Overholser CD. Increased morbidity associated with oral infection in patients with acute nonlymphocytic leukemia. *Oral Surg.* 1981; 51:390.

3.   Sumney DL, Jordan HV, Englander HR. The prevalence of root surface caries in selected populations. *J Periodontol.* 1973; 44:500.

4.   Greensteid G, Berman C, Jaffin R. Chlorhexidine—An adjunct to periodontal therapy. *J Periodontol.* 1986; 57:370.

5.   Overholser Jr CD. Significance of gingivitis in medically compromised patients. *Amer J of Dent.* 1989; 2:295.

6.   Coe FL, Brenner BM. Diseases of the kidney and urinary tract. *Harrison's principals of internal medicine.* Ed 10, New York, McGraw-Hill, 1985.

7.   Cohen SG. Renal disease. *Burket's oral medicine.* Ed 8, Philadelphia, Lippincott Co., 1984.

8.   Greenberg MS, Cohen SG. Oral infection in immunosuppressant renal transplant patients. *Oral Surg.* 1977: 43:879.

9.   Listgarten MA, Slots J, Rosenberg J, Nittein L, Sullivan P, and Older J. Clinical and microbiological characteristics of treated periodontitis patients on maintenance care. *J Periodontol.* 1989; 8:452.

10. Fullerton S. Better non-clinical interaction with geriatric patients. *Dent Mang.* 1990; Jan: 30.

11. Baker KA, Levy SM, Chrischilles EA. Medications with dental significance: usage in a nursing home population. *Special Care in Dent.* 1991; 11:19.

12. Edwards GB, Piepho RW. Pharmacokinetic and pharmocodynamic aspects of geriatric drug therapy. *Gerodontics.* 1985, 1:160.

13. Boyle WD Jr, Via WF, McFall WT Jr. Radiographic analysis of alveolar crest height and ages. *J Periodontol.* 1973; 44:236.

14. Linde J, Scoransky S, Nyman S, Westfelt E, Haffajee A. Effect of age on healing following periodontal therapy. *J Clin Periodontol.* 1985; 12:774.

Chapter 8
Root Caries Risk and Caries Control in Periodontal Patients

Nils Ravald

Periodontal disease and its treatment often cause gingival recession.[1,2,3] The root surfaces are thereby exposed and at risk of caries. Root caries differs from coronal caries due to the different location, anatomy, histology and chemical composition of the tissues. The root cementum and dentin contain about 30% organic material, compared with 2% in the enamel. The "critical pH", the pH at which the root cementum and dentine is dissolved, is 6.0-6.5, compared with 5.2-5.7 for enamel.[4,5] Thus, a wider spectrum of microorganisms might be involved in root caries than in enamel caries.

Diagnosis

Root caries has been described by Banting et al.[6] as a discrete, well-defined and discoloured soft area which an explorer enters easily and displays some resistance to withdrawal. The lesion is located either at the cementoenamel junction or on the root surface. This definition describes a clinically active lesion. As root caries in many instances occurs in inactive or arrested stages[7] i.e., as hard, smooth and dark-brown to black lesions, both active and inactive lesions should be diagnosed and scored. The most frequently used instruments for the diagnosis of root decay are a mirror and explorer. However, excessive probing with explorers should be avoided, since there is a risk of penetration of the superficial layer of root cementum or dentin. If cariogenic microorganisms are introduced into the subsurface layers, the carious lesion might spread in the dentin. It is therefore important to find other methods of diagnosing and measuring root caries activity. Alternative methods have mostly involved analysis of the microbial flora of the root surface plaque[9,10] or indirectly in the saliva.[11] In root caries-active individuals, both plaque and salivary levels and the isolation frequencies of mutans streptococci and lactobacilli have been reported to be elevated compared with inactive individuals. In a recent study,[12] we found significant differences in mutans streptococcus and lactobacillus counts in saliva in untreated periodontal patients with active root caries compared with patients with inactive root caries lesions. Relating the occurrence of microbes in saliva, instead of plaque samples, to root caries activity might be questioned. Lindquist et al.[13] recently showed that the number of mutans streptococci in saliva was correlated with the number of colonised tooth surfaces and the "infection level" of mutans streptococci for individual teeth or groups of tooth surfaces. In patients with exposed root surfaces, positive correlations have been found between the levels of mutans streptococci and lactobacilli in saliva and plaque.[14] Thus, from a clinical point of view, it seems reasonable to use readily obtainable saliva samples, which probably mirror the prevalence of mutans streptococci and lactobacilli on root and coronal surfaces.

Epidemiology

The prevalence of root caries has been studied in selected populations like primitive tribesmen,[15] military personnel, employees and patients in hospitals,[16] institutionalised elderly people[6] and patients treated for periodontal disease.[1,2,3] The prevalence of individuals with one or more decayed or filled root surface varied between 42 and 87%. The highest prevalence has been reported for patients referred for periodontal treatment.[2] However, the prevalence data from these studies are not comparable since the diagnostic criteria and way of reporting root caries differ considerably. In epidemiological studies, the root caries index (RCI) introduced by Katz[17] has been used. In the high-fluoride community of Lordsburg, USA, the mean RCI was as low as 1% in people with a mean age of 43 years.[18] In a Norwegian population of the same age, the RCI was 21%.[19] In elderly individuals, above the mean age of 67 years, RCI scores between 8 and 18% have been reported.[20,21,22] In periodontally treated patients, Keltjens et al.[3] reported an overall mean RCI of 6.3 % in patients with a mean age of 40.6 years. In a recent study,[12] we found a mean of 19 DFS% (decayed filled active or inactive surfaces, related to exposed root surfaces, and expressed as a percentage) in patients, aged between 30 and 78 years (mean age: 52), referred for periodontal treatment. If only active root lesions were included , the score was 6.5 DFS%.

Only a few longitudinal studies of root caries have been reported.[23,24,25] In periodontally treated patients, followed longitudinally for 12 years (unpublished data), we found during the three consecutive 4-year periods a mean of 7, 5 and 10 new DFS% respectively. It thus seems reasonable to believe that patients with periodontal disease, or periodontal patients treated earlier, are at risk for root caries. Although some studies have reported correlations between periodontal disease and root caries,[15,26] there is no evidence that periodontal disease and root caries in humans are caused by the same microorganisms. The risk of root decay should be related to the exposure of root surfaces irrespective of whether the cause is periodontal disease, its treatment or excessive toothbrushing.

The intra-individual distribution of root caries has shown a similar pattern across different studies.[27,28] The most affected teeth are the mandibular molars and the least affected are the mandibular incisors. The mandibular buccal surfaces, especially of the premolar, have shown the highest prevalence of fillings.[28] The prevalence of root decay has been reported to be highest on buccal and approximal surfaces. The lingual surfaces have the least numbers of decayed and filled surfaces. The most prevalent type of caries lesions on root surfaces seems to be secondary caries adjacent to restorations.

Age

The percentage of individuals with root caries and/or fillings has been shown to increase with increasing age.[25,27,29,30] In studies of root caries prevalence, in which root caries has been expressed by root caries index, RCI, the scores have also increased with age. In a recent study in a Swedish population with cohorts categorized by ages 55, 65 and 75 years,[28] the mean RCI was 14%, 16% and 21% respectively. In a 3-year longitudinal study of adults 65 years and older in Iowa, USA, an increased root caries incidence was found with increased age.[25] In patients with treated or untreated periodontal disease[1] an increased prevalence of root caries has been found with increased age. In this patient category, we recently found an increased root caries prevalence up to the age of 65 years and a slight decrease in prevalence, scored in DFS%, thereafter.[12] In a longitudinal study over 12 years (unpublished data), we found an increased root caries incidence during the final 4-year period. The population studied might have been too small to be of general significance, but the findings indicate a correlation between root caries and aging. The increased root caries prevalence and incidence in older populations does not mean an increased correlation between root caries and age *per se*, but it indicates that the risk for root caries increases with age.

Host Factors

When root surfaces are exposed, the possibility of root caries exists. It has been shown that exposure of root surfaces is one main risk factor for root caries.[27] Another factor of importance is that newly exposed root surfaces have a lower content of fluoride.[31] However, other factors, such as the three main factors for enamel caries—the individual, the diet and the microflora—are also of crucial importance for root caries. Illness, medication and changes in social circumstances might significantly affect these factors and thereby be of major importance. There is a large individual variation in external circumstances affecting aging individuals.[32] These factors may be difficult to identify, quantify and influence within the traditional dental sphere.

To solve these problems, dental personnel will have to work in closer cooperation with medical and social service personnel. However, a realistic approach today is to identify and measure factors like salivary conditions, diet, oral hygiene and oral microorganisms, which might be influenced by physical impairments and psychosocial behaviour, but are relatively easily measured by the dental team.

Saliva

The quality and quantity of saliva probably play a major role in the root caries process. With increasing age, structural changes in the salivary glands might occur, but the extent of such changes is not yet completely understood. Healthy elderly people mostly show a normal salivary secretion rate. A decreased mean secretion rate has been reported with increased age. However, low salivary secretion rates among elderly people are in many instances due to medication or ill health.[11,22] A large number of drugs are known to decrease salivary flow. These are to be found among anticholinergics, spasmolytics, analgesics, neuroleptics, antidepressants, antihypertensives, diuretics and antihistamine drugs. Diseases known to decrease salivary flow include rheumatic diseases (Sjögren's syndrome), diabetes, cardiovascular diseases, gastrointestinal diseases and diseases of the nervous system. The salivary buffering capacity is of importance for neutralization of the acid produced by the oral microorganisms. The salivary buffering capacity is correlated with the salivary secretion rate. The prevalence of low buffer capacity, i.e., measurements of pH 4 or less, increases in older age groups, probably due to decreased salivary flow.[11] Other defence mechanisms in the saliva might also be altered in the ill elderly and thereby they would be less effective in preventing caries.[33]

Diet

The importance of the intake frequency of sugar-containing products for caries development was clearly demonstrated in the Vipeholm studies.[34] In periodontally treated and untreated individuals, Hix & O'Leary[1] showed a high correlation between root caries prevalence and intake of fermentable carbohydrates. In our longitudinal study of periodontally treated patients, we also found a positive correlation between intakes of sugar-and starch-containing products and root caries incidence.[24] Other carbohydrates besides sucrose might be of importance for root decay. Starch ingestion yields a milder pH decrease in dental plaque than sucrose, but enough to reach the level for demineralization of root cementum and dentin. In the Vipeholm study, it was shown that new carious lesions developed in some individuals in sucrose-free groups with only limited carbohydrate intake. Starch combined with sucrose seems to be a caries-accelerating factor. The explanation might be that the sugar clearance time is increased by the stickiness of the combination of sucrose and starch. Factors of importance for sugar clearance are the salivary flow, dental status and muscular activity in the masticatory and other muscles associated with the oral cavity. In Swedish hospitalized patients (mean age 80 years) a 3 times longer sugar clearance time was found compared with persons of the same age living at home. Compared with 45-year-old persons, the difference in clearance time was 10 times.[35]

Oral Hygiene

As mentioned before, there is a difference between the pH decrease needed for demineralization of root cementum and dentin compared with enamel. A wider spectrum of microorganisms might therefore be involved in root caries than in coronal caries. In this respect, oral hygiene should be more important for prevention and treatment of root decay. In studies by Axelsson and Lindhe[36,37] it was shown that plaque control and topical application of fluoride was very effective in the prevention of caries and periodontal disease in adults. Data from other studies in periodontally treated or untreated patients revealed no difference in plaque scores between patients with low and high root caries prevalence.[1,2] However, in later studies the importance of oral hygiene has been shown.[24] In a longitudinal study, we have recently found oral hygiene to be one of the most important factors associated with root caries incidence. The effect of oral hygiene in converting clinically active to inactive root lesions has been documented by Nyvad and Fejerskov.[38] They achieved this by meticulous tooth-brushing with fluoride-containing toothpaste. In a recent study in patients referred for treatment of periodontal disease, we have found a significant correlation between active root caries lesions and plaque score.[24]

Microorganisms

Studies of the microbiota of root surface plaque have shown that strictly acidogenic microorganisms such as mutans streptococci and lactobacilli are most likely involved in the root caries process.[9,10] In elderly hospitalised individuals, Ellen et al.[9] showed an increased isolation frequency of mutans streptococci and lactobacilli in root surface plaque from patients who were subsequently found to be root caries active. Moreover, if mutans streptococci alone, or in combination with lactobacilli, were detected on a root surface, the risk for that surface becoming carious increased 3- to 5- fold. In a recent Swedish study,[11] numbers of mutans streptococci and lactobacilli in saliva were found to increase with age. However, it has been shown that root caries can occur in the absence of these microorganisms.[10] Low acid-producing microorganisms like *Actinomyces viscous* and *Actinomyces naeslundii* have been shown to induce periodontal lesions and root caries in animal models.[39,40] In root caries lesions of extracted human teeth[40] and in plaque samples from human carious lesions,[41] *Actinomyces* species have been reported to be the dominant microorganisms. So far, there are no studies showing the significance of *Actinomyces* species in human root caries disease. Their interaction with mutans streptococci and lactobacilli has been shown to be an interesting part of the process.[42] It seems reasonable to believe that other microorganisms besides mutans streptococci and lactobacilli are involved in root caries etiology. However, mutans streptococci and lactobacilli seem to be the most useful "target microorganisms" for monitoring in clinical practice.

Multifactorial Risk Assessment

Swedish scientists and dental clinicians with experience in root caries problems held a consensus conference on root caries in Stockholm in 1990. We concluded that root caries must be considered a multifactorial disease. For root caries to develop there has to be a combination of unfavourable circumstances related to the host, diet and microflora. The following factors were considered to be associated with root caries risk:

—   Newly exposed root surfaces
—   High coronal or root caries incidence or prevalence
—   Low salivary secretion rate
—   Frequent intake of fermentable carbohydrates
—   High numbers of mutans streptococci and lactobacilli
—   High plaque scores
—   Low fluoride exposure

The coexistence of several of these negative factors increases the risk of root decay in the individual patient. Findings from one of our recent studies are in agreement with the conclusions above. We followed a cohort of periodontally treated patients during a 12-year period and monitored the root caries incidence periodically (unpublished data). Factors presumed to influence the root caries process were recorded each 4th year. At the 12-year examination, 27 of the initial 35 patients were examined. Three patients were completely free from new root caries lesions or fillings throughout the 12-year period. Nine patients showed 1-6, six 7-12 and nine greater than 12 new DF root surfaces.

A number of clinical parameters and laboratory tests were recorded and performed during the study. At the 8-year point, the following variables were analyzed and given a "risk border value" as follows: lactobacilli, 10^5 CFU/ml saliva; mutans streptococci, 5×10^5 CFU/ml saliva; plaque score, 50%; salivary secretion rate, 0.7 ml/min; salivary buffering effect, pH 4.5; oral sugar clearance time, 15 min; dietary habit index, 42 intakes of sugar- and starch-containing products per week; and age, 65 years. To show the importance of the variables in the individual patient prospectively, the risk values for patients with 0, 1-5 and more than 5 new DFS% in years 9-12 of the study were grouped together (Table 1).

Table 1 — Number and Distribution of Risk Values for Different Variables at the 8-year Examination in 3 Groups of Subjects with Different New DFS% Scores during Years 9-12

	New DFS%		
	0 (n=6)	1-5 (n=8)	>5 (n=13)
Variables (Risk Border Values)	Number of Subjects		
Age (65 years)			2
Lactobacilli (10^5 CFU/ml)	1	2	6
Mutans streptococci (5×10^5 CFU/ml)	1	1	5
Plaque score (50%)			5
Salivary secretion rate (0.7 ml/min)			1
Salivary buffering effect (pH 4.5)	1	1	2
Oral sugar clearance time (15 min)	1		1
Dietary habit index (42 intakes/week)	1		6
Total	5	4	28

In the total group of 27 patients, 37 risk values were found. The group with >5 new DFS% showed 28 and the groups with 0 and 1-5 new DFS% had 5 and 4 risk values respectively. The most prevalent variables with risk values were salivary lactobacillus count (n=9), salivary mutans streptococcus count (n=7) and dietary habit index (n=7). Such variables probably interact, reflecting an acidogenic environment selective for aciduric bacteria. All risk values for plaque score (n=5) were found in the group with >5 new DFS%. Risk values were simultaneously found for lactobacilli and mutans streptococci in 6 patients, 5 of whom belonged to the group with >5 new DFS%.

The sensitivity, specificity, positive and negative predictive values of selected variables were also calculated. Plaque score and previous root caries incidence (new DFS% in years 5-8) showed the highest sensitivity, both 0.69. The specificity varied between 0.71 (oral sugar clearance time) and 1.0 (salivary secretion rate). High positive predictive values were found for salivary secretion rate (1.0), plaque score (0.90), new DFS% (0.90) and dietary habit index (0.86). In the correlation analysis, significant correlations ($p<0.05$) were found between root caries incidence in years 9-12 and plaque score (0.42), salivary mutans streptococcus count ($r=0.40$), previous root caries incidence ($r=0.39$) and oral sugar clearance time ($r=0.37$). Based on our long-term results, we conclude that the risk of root caries exists in patients treated for periodontal disease. However in a majority of patients this risk is relatively small. In patients with high root caries risk, the number of above threshold values for clinical and laboratory test variables is increased. No single variable is discriminative for development of root caries in all subjects. A combination of above threshold values seems to be crucial for development of root caries. The important variables in this respect differ between individuals.

Individual Risk Evaluation

To identify the individual root caries risk of a patient before periodontal treatment, evaluation of the present root caries risk should be performed. For this purpose, we analyze the patient, the microflora and the diet. Information about environmental factors, *e.g.,* behavioural and socio-economic factors, is also of importance. As these factors are somewhat difficult for the dental team to obtain and especially to influence, the dentist's and dental hygienist's efforts should be focused on the patient's oral problems.

> *The general and dental history* of the patient must include information about general health, medications, smoking habits, dietary habits, dental care and use of fluorides. Special attention should be paid to questions about dryness of the mouth and

perceived dryness, which is often alleviated by sucking on sugar-containing snacks or throat lozenges.

The clinical examination should include information about
- oral mucous membranes
- gingival tissues
- dental plaque (amount and distribution)
- exposure of root surfaces
- prevalence, distribution and quality of previous fillings
- location of coronal and root caries lesions (primary or secondary)
- clinical root caries activity

Saliva samples for determination of secretion rate, buffering effect and content of lactobacilli and mutans streptococci should be taken routinely.

To be able to handle all the data obtained more easily, we have designed a graphic model, useful for the clinician in analyzing the data and as a pedagogic tool for patient information and motivation. An example of an individual root caries risk profile is shown in Figure 1.

Based on information from earlier findings and our longitudinal studies, the following variables and risk border values are suggested to be used as risk indicators for root caries in patients with treated or untreated periodontal disease: age 65 years, root caries incidence >1 lesion/year, plaque score 50%, salivary lactobacillus count 10^5 CFU/ml saliva, mutans streptococcus count 5×10^5 CFU/ml saliva, salivary secretion rate 0.7 ml/min, salivary buffering effect pH 4.5 and >5 intakes per day of sugar- and starch-containing foodstuffs.

Caries Control in Periodontal Patients

Proper diagnosis is a prerequisite for adequate treatment, prophylaxis and prognosis in periodontal patients in relation to both periodontal disease and caries. If the examination shows a low caries activity, the treatment should mainly be symptomatic in character. On the other hand, if the findings indicate future caries risk, every effort should be made to prevent carious lesions, by analysis of cause and prophylactic treatments. The reason why a patient has a low salivary secretion rate should always be analyzed. If the medical problem is already identified by the patient's physician, the possibility of improvement of salivary conditions depends on the type of general disease and the medicine consumed. It is sometimes possible to replace medications which decrease salivary flow. Patients with low salivary flow who have not been examined earlier should be referred for medical examination. Diseases known to decrease salivary flow, e.g., rheumatic disease, diabetes and other hormonal disturbances, should be diagnosed and treated, thereby re-establishing the salivary flow.

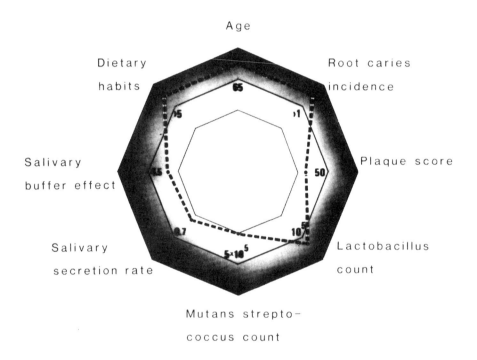

Figure 1 —   *"The root caries risk profile". The threshold risk value of each variable is given. In the profile of this patient, risk values were scored for age, root caries incidence, lactobacillus count and dietary habits.*

Other patients may have vitamin (B-vitamins) or iron deficiency and thus be in need of substitution of these substances.

In addition to general measures, the salivary secretion can be stimulated by chewing a hard, well-composed diet. Individuals with low salivary secretion often use sweets or throat lozenges, which may cause severe root caries within a short time. The sweetener of choice in sweets, chewing-gums, and lozenges for this patient category is xylitol, which is not fermented by mutans streptococci or lactobacilli. Another alternative is fluoride-containing tablets. In Sweden, the fluoride content per tablet differs from 0.25 to 0.75 mg. The total dose of 1.5 mg per day may be divided into 2-6 doses per day, depending on the patient. People with exposed root surfaces should use fluoride toothpaste continuously. After tooth-brushing they should retain toothpaste on their teeth for a time, if possible, and thereby increase the possibility of adding fluoride to the root surfaces. In root caries-active persons individually designed stents for fluoride gel may be the best method of administering fluoride. We recommend 1% sodium fluoride gel for 5 minutes per day as long as the root caries risk exists.

If high numbers of mutans streptococci still exist after oral hygiene improvement, adjustments of fillings or restorations and dietary restrictions, antimicrobial treatment should be performed using 1% chlorhexidine gel in stents. The gel should be applied intensively for 3x5 minutes on two consecutive days or for 5 minutes once each day for 14 days. The former treatment should be performed in a dental office; the latter may be performed at home by patients with a high degree of dexterity and cooperation. The effect of the treatment should be monitored continuously since the number of microbes tends to increase to pretreatment levels within 4-6 months if there are no changes in dietary habits. If the microbial analysis shows low counts of mutans streptococci in combination with medium-high or low sugar intake, intensive professional tooth-cleaning will be the treatment of choice. If possible, the patient should visit a dental hygienist or dental nurse every second month for prophylaxis. In these root caries-active individuals, the fluoride administration is the same (frequent!) regardless of the number of microorganisms.

Conclusions

The risk of root caries in the periodontal patient can be identified at an early stage, before treatment, by means of careful dental and general histories, clinical examination and clinical and laboratory tests. If root caries develops, a causal treatment strategy should be chosen. As the risk of changes in the individual and environmental factors, and thereby the risk of root caries, increases with increased age, elderly patients with exposed root surfaces should pay regular visits to dentists or dental hygienists at least once or twice per year. In diagnosed risk patients, the frequency of dental visits should be 4-6 times per year. In the near future, we should expect a wide range of variation in health status of our patients. More elderly people will be healthy and thereby not at risk for oral disturbances, but still in need of dental prophylaxis. On the other hand, more elderly people will suffer from ill health, which severely affects their oral health, and thereby they will be in need of special attention and care.

Endnotes

1. Hix JO, O'Leary TJ. The relationship between cemental caries, oral hygiene status and fermentable carbohydrate intake. *J Periodontol.* 1976;47:398-04.

2. Ravald N, Hamp S-E. Prediction of root surface caries in patients treated for advanced periodontal disease. *J Clin Periodontol.* 1981;8:400-14.

3. Keltjens HMAM, Schaeken MJM, van der Hoeven JS, Hendriks JCM. Epidemiology of root surface caries in patients treated for periodontal diseases. *Community Dent Oral Epidemiol.* 1988;16:171-4

4. Hoppenbrouwers PMM, Dreissens FCM, Borggreven JMPM. The mineral solubility of human tooth roots. *Arch Oral Biol.* 1987;32:319-22.

5. Katz S, Park KK, Palenik CJ. In-vitro root surface caries studies. *J Oral Med.* 1987;42:40-8.

6. Banting DW, Ellen RP, Fillery ED. Prevalence of root surface caries among institutionalized older persons. *Community Dent Oral Epidemiol.* 1980;8:84-8.

7. Fejerskov O, Luan W-M, Nyvad B, Gadegaard E, Holm-Pedersen P, Budz-Jörgensen E. Root caries in a population of elderly Danes. *J Dent Res.* 1985;64, Spec. Issue: 187, Abstr. no 116.

8. Johansen E, Papas A, Fong W, Olsen TO. Remineralisation of carious lesions in elderly patients. *Geriodontics.* 1987;3:47-50.

9. Ellen RP, Banting DW, Fillery ED. Streptococcus mutans and lactobacillus detection in the assessment of dental root surface caries risk. *J Dent Res.* 1985;64:1245-9.

10. Emilsson C-G, Klock B, Sanford CB. Microbial flora associated with presence of root surface caries in periodontally treated patients. *Scand J Dent Res.* 1988;96:40-9.

11. Fure S, Zickert I. Salivary conditions and cariogenic microorganisms in 55, 65, and 75-year-old Swedish individuals. *Scand J Dent Res.* 1990;98:197-10.

12. Ravald N, Birkhed D. Factors associated with active and inactive root caries in patients with periodontal disease. *Caries Res.* 1991; Accepted for publication.

13. Lindquist B, Emilsson C-G, Wennerholm K. Relationship between mutans streptococci in saliva and their colonization of the tooth surfaces. *Oral Microbiol.* 1989;4:71-6.

14. Fure S, Krasse B. Comparison between different methods for sampling cariogenic microorganisms in persons with exposed root surfaces. *Oral Microbiol Immunol.* 1988;3:173-6.

15. Schamschula RG, Barmes DE, Keyes PH, Gulbinat W. Prevalence and interrelationships of root surface caries in Lufa, Papua, New Guinea. *Community Dent Oral Epidemiol.* 1974;2:295-04.

16. Sumney DL, Jordan HV, Englander HR. The prevalence of root surface caries in selected populations. *J Periodontol.* 1973;44:500-4.

17. Katz RV. Assessing root caries in populations: The evolution of the root caries index. *J Public Health Dent.* 1980;40:7-16.

18. Burt BA, Ismail AI, Eklund SA. Root caries in an optimally fluoridated and a high-fluoride community. *J Dent Res.* 1986;65:1154-8.

19. Gustavsen F, Clive JM, Tveit AB. Root caries prevalence in a Norwegian adult dental patient population. *Gerodontics.* 1988;4:219-23.

20. Forgay MGE, Chebib FS, Knazan YL. Prevalence of root surface caries in a well elderly population. *J Dent Res.* 1986;65, Spec. Issue: 170, Abstr. no 4.

21. Wallace MC, Retief DH, Bradley EL. Prevalence of root caries in a population of older adults. *Gerodontics.* 1988;4:84-9.

22. Kitamura M, Kiyak HA, Mulligan K. Predictors of root caries in elderly. *Community Dent Oral Epidemiol.* 1986;14:34-8.

23. Banting DW, Ellen RP, Fillery ED. A longitudinal study of root caries: baseline and incidence data. *J Dent Res.* 1985;64:1141-4.

24. Ravald N, Hamp S-E, Birkhed D. Long-term evaluation of root surface caries in periodontally treated patients. *J Clin Periodontol.* 1986;13:758-67.

25. Hand JS, Hunt RJ, Beck JD. Coronal and root caries in older Iowans: 36-month incidence. *Gerodontics.* 1988;4:136-9.

26. Locker D, Slade GD, Leake JL. Prevalence of and factors associated with root decay in older adults in Canada. *J Dent Res.* 1989;68:768-72.

27. Katz RV, Hazen SP, Chilton NW, Mumma RD Jr. Prevalence and intraoral distribution of root caries in an adult population. *Caries Res.* 1982;16:265-71.

28. Fure S, Zickert I. Prevalence of root surface caries in 55, 65, and 75-year-old Swedish individuals. *Community Dent Oral Epidemiol.* 1990;18:100-5.

29. Salonen L, Allander L, Bratthall D, Togelius J, Helldén L. Oral health status in an adult Swedish population. Prevalence of caries. *Swed Dent J.* 13:111-23.

30. Vehkalahti M, Rajala M, Tuominen R, Paunio I. Prevalence of root caries in adult Finnish population. *Community Dent Oral Epidemiol.* 1983;11:188-90.

31. Hoppenbrouwers PMM, Dreissens FCM, Borggreven JMPM. The demineralization of human dental roots in the presence of fluoride. *J Dent Res.* 1987;66:1370-4.

32.   Beck JD, Kohout FJ, Hunt RJ, Heckert DA. Root caries: Physical, medical and psychosocial correlates in an elderly population. *Geriodontics*. 1987;3:242-7.

33.   Mandel ID, Wotman S. The salivary secretions in health and disease. *Oral Sciences Rev*. 1976;8:25-47.

34.   Gustavsson BE, Quensel CE, Swenander Lanke L, et al. The Vipeholm dental caries study. *Acta Odontol Scand*. 1954;11:232-64.

35.   Hase JC, Birkhed D, Grennert M-L, Steen B. Salivary glucose clearance and related factors in elderly people. *Gerodontics*. 1987;3:146-50.

36.   Axelsson P, Lindhe J. Effect of controlled oral hygiene procedures on caries and periodontal disease in adults. *J Clin Periodontol*. 1978;5:133-51.

37.   Axelsson P, Lindhe J. Effect of controlled oral hygiene procedures on caries and periodontal disease in adults. Results after 6 years. *J Clin Periodontol*. 1981;8:239-48.

38.   Nyvad B, Fejerskov O. Active root surface caries converted into inactive caries as a response to oral hygiene. *Scand J Dent Res*. 1986;94:281-4.

39.   Jordan HV, Keyes PH, Bellack S. Periodontal lesions in hamsters and gnotobiotic rats infected with actinomyces of human origin. *J Periodont Res*. 1972;7:21-8.

40.   Jordan HV, Hammond BF. Filamentous bacteria isolated from human root surface caries. *Arch Oral Biol*. 1972;17:1333-42.

41.   Syed SA, Loesche WJ, Pape HL Jr, Grenier E. Predominant cultivable flora isolated from human root surface caries plaque. *Infect Immun*. 1975;11:727-31.

42.   Bowden GHW, Ekstrand J, McNaughton B, Challacombe SJ. The association of selected bacteria with the lesions of root surface caries. *Oral Microbiol Immunol*. 1990;5:346-51.

Chapter 9
TMJ and Oral Sensory Disorders in Older Adults

Marc W. Heft

Introduction

As has been reviewed in the previous chapters, there are increased medical problems with age. Many of these disorders have an impact on daily functioning and are underscored by a multitude of physical symptoms in the elderly. For example, these may be from decreased locomotion due to a painful arthritic knee, or decreased visual accommodation with presbyopia requiring the use of reading glasses to assist in near vision. Of particular interest are the painful maladies observed in the aged because the symptom of pain oftentimes signals tissue damage stimuli; this can have potentially dire consequences for the integrity and functioning of the individual.

Decline in sensory function has been thought to be a concomitant of the normal aging process. While the evidence strongly supports this view of age-related declines for vision, audition, and olfaction (smell), the findings are more equivocal for touch, temperature sense, taste, and pain.[1] Many of the conflicting results in the experimental literature in this area reflect differences in paradigm (for example, some experiments assess thresholds for pain, while others assess stimuli that evoke graded painful sensations) and differences in the painful stimuli used (for example, some experiments have used noxious heat, others have used electrocutaneous shock, and others have used ischemic pain produced by a tourniquet applied to the arm or leg). Recent studies by Harkins et al.[2] and Heft et al[3,4] employing painful thermal stimuli to the arm and face, respectively, reported no differences in pain perception with age.

The belief that the sensory experience of pain is changed with aging has been supported by clinical evidence. Numerous reports have documented that various conditions such as myocardial infarction or appendicitis, which are normally associated with pain in younger individuals, may not be associated with pain or pain of a similar magnitude in an older individual.[1,5] However, the disease may present with symptoms that include behavioural changes (such as confusion, fatigue, or restlessness) or the pain symptom may be embedded within the concurrent presentation of multiple chronic diseases within an elderly individual.

Several painful conditions occur more commonly in older individuals. Clinical features of several of these conditions suggest that they are associated with changes in sensory processing in that pain is elicited by non-noxious stimulation (light touch or pressure). Most notable among these are trigeminal neuralgia, post-herpetic neuralgia, and glossodynia.

Trigeminal Neuralgia (see ref. 6 for a review): Trigeminal neuralgia, or tic douloureux, is a syndrome of the face characterized by: 1. severe paroxysms of pain elicited by a non-noxious stimulus such as light touch applied to a specific location on the face (trigger point), 2. occurrence of a severe, abrupt paroxysm of "electric-like" pain, unilaterally within a division of the trigeminal nerve (primarily the second and third divisions, maxillary and mandibular), and 3. the paroxysm lasts anywhere from several seconds to several minutes with a pain-free period between attacks of pain. The disorder presents mainly in individuals greater than 50 years of age, with women afflicted somewhat more often than men. The disorder is thought to have both a peripheral component (triggered by a somatosensory stimulus) and a central component (non-noxious stimuli are eliciting pain). The treatments include surgical interventions (e.g., radiofrequency thermal coagulation, which selectively destroys the peripheral sensory nerves, and microvascular decompression of the trigeminal root) and pharmacological interventions (phenytoin, carbamazepine, and baclofen).

Post-Herpetic Neuralgia (see ref. 7 for a review): Postherpetic neuralgia (PHN) is a pain syndrome caused by herpes zoster, and it is related to a reactivation of a varicella zoster virus (chicken pox) contracted in childhood. The acute herpes zoster infection begins with pain and dysesthesia in the afflicted dermatome before the eruption of vesicles. The vesicles scab in one week and heal within one month. "Postherpetic neuralgia" refers to the pain which persists after the acute infection has run its course. Older patients and immunosuppressed individuals are more likely to develop the condition, which suggests that decreased immune function is a risk factor for the disorder. While it has been reported that PHN afflicts females more often than males, Watson[7] has suggested that the reported prevalence reflects the higher percentage of females in the older age groups. PHN afflicts mainly the trigeminal and thoracic segmental distributions and is usually unilateral in presentation. The condition is characterized by burning pain within the affected dermatome, and there are sensory deficits marked by reduced or absent appreciation of light touch or pinprick. The treatments of choice are principally pharmacological, and they include tricyclic antidepressants, tricyclic antidepressants with neuroleptics, anticonvulsants, and capsaicin.

Glossodynia (Burning Mouth Syndrome) (see ref. 8 for a review): Glossodynia or Burning Mouth Syndrome is an intraoral painful disorder which afflicts primarily postmenopausal females. It is characterized by sensations of hyperesthesia, dysesthesia, or allodynia afflicting the tongue and other soft tissues of the mouth. The presumed etiology has included: 1. local (peripheral) factors (foliate papillitis, galvanism, dentures, ischemia, neuropathies), 2. xerostomia, 3. systemic factors, including: hormonal factors (menopause), nutritional deficiencies, and systemic disease (e.g., diabetes), and 4. miscellaneous factors, including psychological factors. Grushka[8] has suggested that there are peripheral changes in somatosensory processing with this condition. Treatment approaches have varied with the presumed etiology of the symptoms, and they include replacement of dental restorations, local anaesthetic blocks, nutritional supplements, as well as medical management of systemic disease (such as diabetes).

Another set of painful conditions of interest in the dental literature has been the temporomandibular disorders, although recent evidence has suggested that this is not the case. Two putative risk factors that were thought to support the increased prevalence of these disorders with age are increased rates of tooth loss (and edentulousness) and the increased prevalence of arthritis with age. The term "temporomandibular disorders" refers to a class of painful disturbances of the masticatory system marked by symptoms of temporomandibular joint pain on function or pain in the face, including the preauricular area, and the presence of one or more of the following signs: limitation in the range of motion of the mandible on function, deviation of the mandible on function, or noises in the TMJ.

Patients seeking care for temporomandibular disorders are typically females between the ages of 20-40 years.[9-15] Epidemiological studies have reported that there are no gender differences in signs and symptoms in non-patient populations.[16-22] Reports from studies assessing age-differences in TMD have provided conflicting results.[16,17,19-29] Part of the confusion in comparing survey results is that these studies have typically employed three different data collection methods. The most objective and consistent data across studies are derived from direct clinical measurement of such signs as mouth opening, deviation, or the presence of TMJ noise (without regard to presence on opening or closing, or the quality of the sound). The clinical measures are in contrast to the less objective data obtained from mailed questionnaires and anamnestic studies (clinical questionnaires), both of which require subjective assessments of functioning or reports of symptoms.

Some studies have attempted to compare qualitative measures of function with directly measurable clinical assessments of function. For example, interincisal opening of less than 40 mm has been considered an indicator of decreased function. It is directly measurable and shows a reasonable degree of reproducibility among examiners.[30] Qualitative data such as an affirmative response to the question "Do you have difficulty in opening your mouth to eat an apple?" reflect not only a level of functioning, but also a self-assessment of that functioning. These data are clearly not the same. We would expect that there are individuals who report opening sufficiently well but who are unable to open 40 mm, and vice versa, there are individuals who complain of being unable to open sufficiently but who exhibit an opening of 40+ mm. The subject's judgment reflects ability and performance, but also requires an evaluation that can be influenced by psychological factors. Even for one of the signs, joint noises, which we would expect to have the greatest agreement between clinical observation (sign) and patient report (symptom), the reports indicate a marked discordance (see ref. 31 for review of this issue).

In a review of TMD epidemiology studies, Heft[24] reported that three clinical measures of mandibular function were the most objective (i.e., showed the most consistency across studies). The greatest interexaminer agreement was for mouth opening, presence of temporomandibular joint noises (without regard to classification as click, crepitation, or grating), and presence of deviation of the mandible on opening or closing. Greene and Marbach[32] criticized the inclusion of the different qualities of joint noises under the same heading, since presumably the joint sounds can arise from different underlying pathologies. Heft suggested that the ambiguity in reporting joint sounds might account for the broad range in reported prevalence (27-60% for the elderly, 14-51% for younger individuals). This contrasts with decreased mouth opening (1-20% for the elderly, 3.5%-5% for younger individuals), which employed a stricter measurement criterion.

In reviewing the studies of age differences in the occurrence of TMD signs and symptoms, Heft[24] noted that two of the studies[17,19] included only elderly subjects and a third study[16] suggested that the observed age differences were attributable to denture-related problems. In considering research needs in this area, Heft emphasized that there was a need for standardization of clinical, questionnaire, and anamnestic data collection methods to allow for meaningful comparisons both in longitudinal studies (to assess time and treatment related changes in the signs and symptoms) and across studies.

The purpose of the ensuing studies was to assess the occurrence of signs and symptoms of TMD in non-health-care-seeking individuals (not patients) using a standardized data collection methodology.[24] Based on the preliminary study, it was decided to consider five measures of three signs and two symptoms of TMD in the clinical study. The three signs: mouth opening, presence of temporomandibular joint noises, and deviation of the mandible on opening or closing were directly observable by the trained examiner. The two pain symptom reports were responses to anamnestic queries.

Methods

Samples:
Subjects in the studies included four groups. The first group included participants in the Baltimore Longitudinal Study of Aging (BLSA), based in the intramural program of the National Institute on Aging, at the Gerontology Research Centre.[33,34] This sample includes 144 consecutive participants in the oral physiology component of the BLSA. The community-dwelling volunteers

ranged in age from 19-86 years (mean age of 56 years, 57% males). The subjects were examined by the author. Two additional groups of predominantly older volunteers were examined at two senior activity centres in Alachua County, Florida using the same data collection methodology.[35,36] The first senior centre included primarily Caucasians (N=71, 38% male, mean age= 72.1 yrs). The second senior centre constituted a primarily Black sample (N=73, 45% male, mean age=73.6 yrs). Data were collected from two examiners at each site who were trained and standardized in the clinical data collection procedure.

Procedure:

All clinical data were collected with the subject seated in either a dental chair (BLSA) or straight back chair (senior centres). The clinical data were collected as described:

Signs:

Temporomandibular Joint Noises. The presence or absence of joint noise was the measure of interest. No attempt was made to further classify noises as clicks, crepitation or grating. Subjects were instructed to open and close their mouths. Notation was made as to the presence of an audible sound (yes or no), when it was present (opening, closing, or both), and where it was present (left, right, or both). In the event that a subject reported a noise when none was heard by the examiner, manual palpation of the temporomandibular joint was employed to corroborate the patient's report (however for this analysis, only the examiner noted finding was used).

Deviation. The subject was instructed to open and close his/her mouth. The examiner noted whether the mandible shifted upon opening or closing of the mouth. Gross measure of shifting of the mandible was noted, as were when it occurred (opening, closing, or both), and to which side it occurred. No attempt was made to measure the amount of shift. For analysis, only the presence or absence of shift was considered.

Mouth Opening. Subjects were asked to open their mouths maximally. The distance between the midlines of the maxillary and mandibular central incisors was measured with a millimetre rule. If the patient was missing these teeth, distances were measured from the denture teeth (no patients were missing teeth without having replacements). No adjustment was made in the opening measure to correct for overbite and overjet relations. The dependent measure was opening in mm.

Symptoms:

Pain on Function. Subjects were asked to open their mouths maximally as in the opening procedure and then to close. They were then instructed to move their mandible laterally from side to side. Subjects were then queried about the presence of pain on these movements. The presence of pain on any movement constituted a yes response.

History of Head, Face, or Ear Pain. The report of the occurrence of head, face, or ear pain was elicited upon clinical history. Additional information was sought upon whether the individual acted on the symptom (for example, sought care or took medication); however, this information was not included in the present analysis.

Results and Discussion

The results of this study are shown in Table 1. The Baltimore Longitudinal Study (BLSA) participants (43% female) are divided into two groups: "young", connoting those below the mean age of 56 years, and "old", connoting those greater than 56 yrs. The "TMD patients" included 48 consecutive TMD patients seen by the author in a pain clinic environment. The TMD patient data are provided as a comparison with regard to the *a priori* signs and symptoms of TMD. These patients were characterized as chronic pain patients in that their pain had persisted for at least 6 months in duration and patients were referred to the facility from their attending clinician. The patients were 85% female and the mean age was 41 years. The Florida-Caucasian sample was 62% female with a mean age of 72.1 years, and the Florida-Black sample was 55% female with a mean age of 73.6 years. The Florida samples were somewhat older than the BLSA and TMD samples, and the percentage of female subjects in the samples was greater than BLSA but less than the TMD patients.

The occurrence of the three signs are fairly consistent across the three elderly samples, ranging from 22% to 34% for temporomandibular joint noises, 10% to 42% for deviation, and 13 to 33% for opening less than 40 mm. The TMD patient group, however, had a significantly higher occurrence of joint noises (65%). As reported previously,[24] the younger BLSA individuals had a slightly greater mouth opening than the older BLSA participants.

With regard to the symptoms of TMD, there was greater agreement among these groups than has been reported in the literature. Those reporting pain on function ranged from 3% to 8%, in contrast to the 42% prevalence among the TMD patients. For those reporting a history of head, face, or ear pain, the occurrences range from 20% to 27%, which is considerably less than the 90% prevalence reported by the TMD patients (which is what would be expected—i.e., most TMD patients are seeking care for head, face, or ear pain). Of the elderly subjects who report a history of face pain, 41% of the BLSA old, 73% of the Florida- Caucasian, and 76% of the Florida- Black reported seeking care for the condition. In contrast, 95% of the BLSA- young reported seeking care for face pain. However, these data suggest that relatively high percentages of young and elderly individuals who report face pain do indeed seek care for the condition, which is consistent with the report by Harkins et al.[37]

Table 1 — Prevalence of Selected Signs and Symptoms of Temporomandibular Disorders in Patient and Non-Patient Samples*

	BLSA young	BLSA old	TMD patients	Florida — Caucasian	Florida — Black
Signs:					
Noise	32	34	65	33	22
Deviation	36	38	38	42	10
Opening < 40 mm	5	13	33	26	33
Symptoms:					
Pain on Function	8	5	42	3	3
History of Head, Face, or Ear Pain	20	27	90	29	23
* As percentage of sample					

Of further interest is the relationship between the *a priori* signs and symptoms of temporomandibular disorders. History of head, face, or ear pain is the most common presenting symptom of TMD. The relationship between this symptom and having at least one of the two signs, deviation of the mandible on function or joint noises, is shown in Table 2. Many clinicians consider the latter sign as an indication of pathological change in the temporomandibular joint. The prevalence of having at least one sign ranges from 30% to 57% for the non-patient groups, as compared with 73% for the TMD patient group. However, having at least one sign was not strongly associated with the presence of the symptom in the non-patient samples. Amongst the TMD patient group, 65/73 or 89% of patients with either sign have the head pain symptom. In contrast, only 33% of BLSA-young, 21% of BLSA-old, 39% of Florida-Caucasian, and 40% of Florida-Black show this association, or greater than half (60% to 79% of the elderly individuals with presence of the *a priori* signs do not have TMD symptoms). A X^2 analysis failed to establish an association between these signs and symptoms and further failed to find significant differences between the young and elderly non-patients.

**Table 2 — Relationship Between the Presence of Either
of Two Signs* of Temporomandibular Disorders
and the History of Head, Ear, or Face Pain***

	BLSA young	BLSA old	TMD patients	Florida — Caucasian	Florida — Black
Pain and ≥1 sign	17	12	65	22	12
No pain and ≥1 sign	34	44	8	35	18
Prevalence of ≥1 sign	51	56	73	57	30

* Either deviation or joint noise
** As percentage of sample

Thus, while various painful conditions such as trigeminal neuralgia and postherpetic neuralgia are diseases of increasing age, temporomandibular disorders do not appear to be diseases of aging.

Endnotes

1. Harkins, S.W. Pain in the elderly. In: Dubner, R., Gebhart, G.F., Bond, M.R. eds. *Proceedings of the vth world congress on pain.* New York: Elsevier, 1988:355-367.

2. Harkins, S.W., Price, D.D., Martelli, M. Effects of age on pain perception: thermonociception. *Journal of Gerontology.* 1986; 41:58-63.

3. Heft, M.W., O'Brien, R., O'Brien, K. Consistency in judgments of thermal stimuli between young and elderly subjects [Abstract]. *J Dent Res.* 1991; 70 (Special Issue): 365.

4. Heft, M.W., O'Brien, R.G., Cooper, B.Y., O'Brien, K. Age effects in the perception of noxious heat stimuli to the lip and chin [Abstract]. *Abstracts of the American Pain Society Ninth Annual Scientific Meeting.* 1990: 26.

5. Butler, R.N., Gastel, B. Care of the aged: perspectives on pain and discomfort. In: Ng, L.K.Y., Bonica, J.J. eds. *Pain, discomfort and humanitarian care.* New York: Elsevier, 1980: 297-311.

6. Fromm, G.H. Trigeminal neuralgia and related disorders. In: Portenoy, R.K., ed. *Neurologic clinics.* 1989; 7(2): 305-319.

7. Watson, C.P.N. Postherpetic neuralgia. In: Portenoy, R.K., ed. *Neurologic clinics.* 1989;7(2): 231-248.

8. Grushka, M. Clinical features of burning mouth syndrome. *Oral Surg Oral Med Oral Pathol.* 1987; 63:30-36.

9. Carraro, J.J., Cafesse, R.G. Albano, E.A. Temporomandibular joint syndrome. *Journal of Prosthetic Dentistry.* 1969; 28:54-62.

10. Franks, A.S.T. The social character of temporomandibular dysfunction. *Dental Practitioner and Dental Record.* 1964; 15:94-100.

11. Helkimo, M. Epidemiological surveys of dysfunction of the masticatory system. In: Zarb, G.A., Carlsson, G.E. eds. *Temporomandibular joint: function and dysfunction.* St. Louis: CV Mosby, 1979:175-192.

12. Helöe, B., Helöe, L.A. Frequency and distribution of myofascial pain dysfunction syndrome in a population of 25 year olds. *Community Dentistry and Oral Epidemiology.* 1979; 7:357-360.

13. Perry, H.T. The symptomology of the temporomandibular joint disturbances. *Journal of Prosthetic Dentistry.* 1969; 9:288-298.

14. Schwartz, L.L., Cobin, H.P. Symptoms associated with the temporomandibular joint. *Oral Surgery.* 1957; 10:339-344.

15. Thompson, H. Mandibular joint pain. a survey of 100 treated cases. *British Dental Journal.* 1959; 107: 243-245.

16. Agerberg, G., Carlsson, G.E. Functional disorders of the masticatory system. i. Distribution of symptoms according to age and sex as judged from investigation by questionnaire. *Acta Odontologica Scandinavica.* 1972; 30:597-613.

17. Agerberg, G., Osterberg, T. Maximal mandibular movements and symptoms of mandibular dysfunction in 70 year old men and women. *Swedish Dental Journal.* 1974; 67:1-17.

18. Hansson, T., Nilner, M. A study of the occurrence of symptoms of diseases of the tmj, masticatory musculature, and related structures. *Journal of Oral Rehabilitation.* 1975; 2:239-243.

19. Hansson, T., Oberg, T. En kliniskt-bett-fysiologisk undersokning av 67-aringer i dalby. *Tandlakartidn.* 1971; 63:650-655.

20. Helkimo, M. Studies on function and dysfunction of the masticatory system. iv. Age and sex distribution of symptoms of dysfunction of the masticatory system in Lapps in the north of Finland. *Acta Odontologica Scandinavica.* 1974; 37:255-267.

21. Ingervall, B., Hedegard, B. Subjective evaluation of functional disturbances of the masticatory system in young Swedish men. *Community Dentistry and Oral Epidemiology.* 1974; 2:149-152.

22. Molin, C. Carlsson, G.E., Friling, B., Hedegard, B. Frequency of symptoms of mandibular dysfunction in young Swedish men. *Journal of Oral Rehabilitation.* 1976; 3:9-18.

23. Gross, A., Gale, E. A prevalence study of the clinical signs associated with the mandibular dysfunction syndrome. *JADA.* 1983; 107:932-936.

24. Heft, M.W. Prevalence of tmj signs and symptoms in the elderly. *Gerodontology.* 1984; 3:125-130.

25. Helöe, B., Helöe, L.A. The occurrence of tmj-disorders in an elderly population as evaluated by recording of "subjective" and "objective" symptoms. *Acta Odontologica Scandinavica.* 1978; 36:3-9.

26. Norheim, P.W., Dahl, B.L. Some self-reporting symptoms of temporomandibular dysfunction in a population in northern Norway. *Journal of Oral Rehabilitation.* 1978; 5:63-68.

27. Osterberg, T., Carlsson, G.E. Symptoms and signs of mandibular dysfunction in 70-year-old men and women in Gothenburg, Sweden. *Community Dentistry and Oral Epidemiology.* 1979; 7:315-321.

28. Rieder, C.E., Martinoff, J.T., Wilcox, S.A. The prevalence of mandibular dysfunction. part i: Sex and age distribution of related signs and symptoms. *Journal of Prosthetic Dentistry.* 1983; 50:81-88.

29. Solberg, W.K., Woo, M.W., Houston, J.B. Prevalence of mandibular dysfunction in young adults. *JADA.* 1979; 98:25-34.

30. Dworkin, S.F., LeResche, L., DeRouen, T., Von Korff, M. Assessing clinical signs of temporomandibular disorders: reliability of clinical examiners. *J Prosthet Dent*. 1990; 63:574-579.

31. Dworkin, S.F., Huggins, K.H., LeResche, L., Von Korff, M., Howard, J., Truelove, E., Sommers, E. Epidemiology of signs and symptoms in temporomandibular disorders: clinical signs in cases and controls. *JADA*. 1990; 120:273-281.

32. Green, C.S., Marbach, J.J. Epidemiological studies of mandibular dysfunction: a critical review. *Journal of Prosthetic Dentistry*. 1982; 48:184-190.

33. Baum, B.J. Characteristics of participants in the oral physiology component of the Baltimore longitudinal study of aging. *Community Dentistry and Oral Epidemiology*. 1981; 9:128-134.

34. Stone, J., Norris, A. Activities and attitudes of participants in the Baltimore longitudinal study. *Journal of Gerontology*. 1966; 21:575-580.

35. Clark, L.L., Heft, M.W. Signs and symptoms of temporomandibular disorders among an ambulatory elderly sample [Abstract]. *J Dent Res*. 1987; 66:187.

36. Malone, B.L., Vallerand, W. and Heft, M.W. Signs and symptoms of temporomandibular disorders (tmd) in an ambulatory black elderly sample [Abstract]. *J Dent Res*. 1988; 67: 176.

37. Harkins, S.W., Bush, F.M., Price, D.D. The effects of age on presentation of orofacial pain: more absence than presence [Abstract]. *J Dent Res*. 1991; 70 (Special Issue): 365.

Part 2: Opinion

Chapters 10–17 are multi-authored chapters titled "opinion" because they are based on discussions and debate in small workshop groups. The authors represent the panelists, the first author being the panel leader, who presented a summary of the group's activities and recommendations to the plenary session on the second day of the symposium. Because the group leaders and panelists were given independence and free choice in designing approaches to lively interchange, the formats of the chapters are diverse. Some appear as formal multi-authored manuscripts; others appear as detailed outlines. As there really is very little peer-reviewed, concrete information specific to periodontal care for older adults, the groups were charged with the responsibility to generate a list of recommendations of needs and suggested improvements. All of the authors have first-hand experience in their assigned topic fields. While stylistically different, a pattern of guidelines for periodontal care and concerns emerges.

Chapter 10
Periodontics — Restorative Treatment Planning for Older Adults: Services for Dependents in Collective Living Centres

Adrianne M. Schmitt, Roy S. Feldman, and Hardy Limeback

The 20 participants of the discussion group comprised dental hygienists, general dentists and periodontists, most of whom had experience working with older adults residing in collective living centres.

As a starting point for discussion, the following ideas were presented by the panel leaders:

1. Recent data collected from a study of the residents of a group of homes for the aged in Toronto, summarised in Table 1, are representative of the state of dental health of the people in many such institutions. This differs from the statistics of just a few years ago, when percentages of residents with teeth ranged from 19% to 30% (Table 2).[1-5] Along with this increased number of people with natural or restored teeth comes a need for greater availability of professional dental care and an increased demand for a dramatic improvement in daily oral hygiene.

2. Experience in the study of masticatory efficiency with various replacements for lost natural dentitions indicate that function is best preserved with fixed partial dentures, and least preserved with removable appliances. Experimental models for patterns of mastication show complete pulverization of food particles within approximately 40 chewing strokes for all dentitions studied. Therefore, while evidence has been presented to document no difference in chewing efficiency in overdentures over time in a test using 80 chewing strokes, the prolonged testing may obscure important clinical differences in function. Alveolar bone, however, seems to be preserved during the first year after extraction when mandibular canine teeth are retained as overdenture abutments. In summary, the natural dentition appears to benefit greatly the clinical situation in many ways: patient performance may be enhanced, psychologic support is maintained as the patient feels that teeth are preserved, alveolar bone may be more resistant to resorption, and prosthodontic management may be facilitated.[6-12]

3. Older patients have been, and are being, treated with osseointegrated implants in an attempt to alleviate the problems they have with wearing complete dentures. It has been demonstrated that the periodontal indices recorded around Brånemark implants do not correlate well with the state of integration of the implants.[13, 14]

4. Although we know that oral hygiene for those people in collective centres is ultimately the responsibility of the caregiver, we must recognize the difficulties they face. For instance, there are those residents who, to say the least, are resistive. In response to an attempt to have their teeth brushed, they bite and spit or scream or lash out. Is it the duty of the caregiver to face this abuse? Is it within the rights of the patient to decline oral hygiene? Is it within the rights of the patient to decline dental treatment?

Table 1 — Dental Health in a Home for the Aged

Total number of residents in study	2400
Number of dentate residents	1128
Mean age	80 years
Female/male ratio	3:1
% with natural teeth	47
Mean # of natural teeth	11
Mean oral hygiene index	4.2 (1 is 'good', 5 is 'none')
Caries progression	1.8 new lesions/person/year
Tooth loss	0.6 teeth/person/year

To begin the discussion, the members of the group were polled in order to create a list of the various treatment modalities available to the older adult patient in a collective living centre. These are listed in order of presentation in Table 3. As the list was being produced, it became obvious that the main issue was not the treatments available, but rather an overall sense of complete frustration with the *system*. The dentists are capable of carrying out the treatment, but can the system—the patient, the administration and the caregiving personnel cope with it? And even more than just coping, can the *system* cooperate and provide the necessary assistance and support to allow the dental personnel to provide good and lasting dental treatment so that the residents will have clean, healthy, comfortable and functional mouths.

Table 2 — Rates of 'Dentulism' in the Institutionalised Elderly

Year of Study	City	% Dentulous	Age Group	Reference
1969	London	23	50-59	Martinello, Leake[1]
1969	Toronto	19	50-59	Lightman et al.[2]
1976	Chatham	24	50+	Martinello[3]
1982	East York	24	62-99	Leake and Howley[4]
1985	Scarborough	30	60-90	McIntyre et al.[5]

To make use of the experience and talents of the group, the Delphi method was employed to develop a list of the categories of personnel involved in the oral care of people living in institutional settings. The responsibilities, the concerns and the worries and the frustrations about each of these are enumerated under the appropriate heading. They are listed as expressed by the members of the discussion group and in the order in which they were presented.

Table 3 — Appropriate Treatment Modalities

No treatment
Preventive fluoride only
Implants
Extractions
Endodontics
Plaque control
Antibiotics
Restorations
Prosthetics

Providers Involved in Oral Care of Residents of Institutions

Dentist
    (i)   first function is diagnosis of oral disease
    (ii)   are seen or made to feel to be intruders in hospital
    (iii)   constant lack of funds
    (iv)   M.D. is required to approve treatment
    (v)   need more knowledge of medical conditions
    (vi)   education of dental students is not targeted to needs of the older patient
    (vii) lack of cooperation
    (viii) frustration surrounding points (ii) to (vii).

Dental Hygienist
    (i)   training is weak in geriatrics
    (ii)   a major role is diagnosis of pathologic disorders
    (iii)   need better understanding of work in a hospital or seniors' residence
    (iv)   need to train other personnel caring for geriatric residents
    (v)   require more family support for oral hygiene.

Dental Assistant
    (i)   require more specialized training in dealing with older patients
    (ii)   nursing attendants better trained in handling patient but are not interested in assisting the dentist.

Denture Therapist
    (i)   worry regarding diagnostic ability
    (ii)   should not be making partial dentures
    (iii)   need a better defined role in providing prosthodontic support.

Nurses and Nursing Attendant
    (i)   in the present system, the nurse recognizes the dental complaint—refers to physician who refers to the dentist
    (ii)   needs to expand diagnostic skills to improve the potential to contribute to the evaluation/diagnosis or oral problems
    (iii)   needs to appreciate the significance of oral problems in patient management
    (iv)   often has no interest
    (v)   no knowledge of dental matters
    (vi)   no time to include proper oral care

(vii)   often have different priorities that do not include oral care

(viii)   is the daily provider of dental care.

Physician

(i)   controls the activities of the dentist

(ii)   is uninformed of dentist's ability

(iii)   is uninformed as to dental needs of patient

(iv)   too busy for dental consideration

(v)   needs more sophistication in oral diagnostic skills.

Administration

(i)   do not want dental personnel in the system

(ii)   lack of follow-up

(iii)   resists administrative creativity

(iv)   is responsible for the 'physical plant'

(v)   needs to appreciate the therapeutic benefit to be derived from geriatric dentistry

(vi)   potential for improvement of patient health should be assessed by cost/benefit methodology to establish rationale for inclusion of dental therapy.

Corporations

(i)   need better technology directed to geriatric population

(ii)   educational materials directed toward the elderly

(iii)   need to understand the developing market for products.

Family

(i)   need education regarding dental needs.

Government

(i)   provides the funds for medical and dental services

(ii)   needs better understanding regarding the need for dentist and oral care in each residence

(iii)   needs better legislation regarding dental and oral care facilities.

Although the list was long and complex, two themes were common to all categories. One theme was the need for more, better and continued education, for the dental professionals, the medical professionals, government, families and the business community. The other was an overwhelming sense of frustration with the lack of cooperation among the other 'role players'.

To be sure, the constant lack of funds is an important concern, but the education and cooperation and coordination of the personnel involved are the paramount issues. Without a willingness to be supportive, to understand, and to assist each other, all these 'role players' who comprise the caregivers for the dependent elderly will not succeed in providing adequate dental care for them.

Endnotes

1. Martinello, B.P. and Leake, J.L. Oral health status in the three London, Ontario, homes for the aged. *Can Dent Assoc J.* 1971, 37(11) 429-32.
2. Ligthtman, I., Thompson, G.W. and Granger, R.M. Denture needs of a group of Toronto aged. *Can Dent Assoc J.* 1969, 35 40-4.
3. Martinello, B.P. Oral health assessment of residents of a Chatham, Ontario, home for the aged. *Can Dent Assoc J.* 1976, 42 405-8.
4. Leake, J.L. and Howley, T.P Dental health status of residents of a Toronto home for the aged. *Session No.3004, American Public Health Association meeting.* Montreal, Quebec, 1982.
5. McIntyre, R.T. Dental health status and treatment needs of seniors in Scarborough nursing homes and homes for the aged. Scarborough, Ontario: *Health Department.* 1985.
6. Feldman, R.S. and Chauncey, H.H. Aging and mastication changes in performance and swallowing threshold with natural dentition. *J Am Geriatrics Soc.* 1980, 38 97-103.
7. Chauncey, H.H., Kapur, K.K. and Feldman, R.S. Altered masticatory function and perceptual estimates of chewing experience. *Spec Care Dent.* 1981, 1 250-255.
8. Wayler, A.H., Kapur, K.K., Feldman, R.S. and Chauncey, H.H. Effect of age and dentition status on measures of food acceptability. *J Gerontol.* 1982, 37 294-299.
9. Feldman, R.S., Alman, J.E., Muench, M.E. and Chauncey, H.H. Longitudunal stability and masticatory function in human dentition. *J Gerodont.* 1984, 3(2) 107-113.
10. Rissin, L., Feldman, R.S. Kapur, K.K. and Chauncey, H.H. Peridontal status of fixed and removable partial denture abutment teeth: a six year report. *J Pros Dent.* 1985, 4(4) 461-469.
11. van Waas, M.A.G., Jonkman, R.E.G., Kalk, W. and Plooy, J. Alveolar bone reduction with immediate dentures versus overdentures. *J Dent Res.* 1991, 70 2345 (ABS).
12. Kalk, W., Plooy, J., van Waas, M.A.G. and Jonkman, R.E.G. Chewing efficiency with immediate dentures versus overdentures. *J Dent Res.* 1991, 70 2344 (ABS).
13. Zarb, G.A. and Schmitt, A. Terminal dentition in elderly patients. *Int Dent J.* 1990, 40 67-73.
14. Apse, P., Zarb, G.A., Schmitt, A. and Lewis, D. The longitudinal effectiveness of osseointegrated dental implants. The Toronto Study: Peri-implant Mucosal Response. *Int J of Perio and Rest Dent.* 1991, 11 94-111.

Chapter 11
Bearing the Cost of Long-term Periodontal Care: Public, Private, and Third Party Options

James L. Leake, James D. Beck, Sidney Golden, and David M. Kogon

To consider this topic, the group of panel members included a professor of community dentistry who is director of a dental public health unit in Canada, a professor of dental ecology and epidemiology from the U.S.A., a private practitioner specialist and teacher in periodontics, and a representative of a private company which analyzes the private insurance sector. Their different experiences and diverse orientations to the problem of dental health funding for older adults led to a list of recommendations for consideration.

Dr. Golden, the private practitioner/teacher, based his contribution on a videotape of structured interviews with three of his patients and similar interviews with patients who were not included in the videotape. These patients were obviously "affluent" and already motivated to seek specialist care long-term. They might be thought of as "conservative" members of society. All three valued their teeth highly. One pointed to the potential emotional loss associated with tooth loss; another rated retention of teeth second only to eyesight. They agreed that they would pay a considerable sum of money to keep their teeth, and they felt that the contribution of a natural dentition to their appearance was very important. They would favour continuing care with their preferred provider. Their opinions regarding the costs of dental care were as follows:

— Two suggested that dentists should give a fee reduction of 25-35% to older adults.
— One suggested that dentists should not have to make the assessment of who deserved lower costs.
— All three felt that insurance would help and that they would be willing to pay premiums of an unstated amount.
— All three felt that Government should cover this as part of its social benefits.

David Kogon presented a review of the perspectives of the dental insurers in Ontario. Some salient points of his review were:

— The cost of privately insured plans is continuing to rise faster than the rate of the fee increases.
— Costs of periodontal care are rising rapidly, sometimes as much as 30-60% from one year to the next.
— Insurers lack the information needed to properly adjudicated claims for periodontal care, i.e., assure the plan sponsors

(employer and employee groups) that all services paid for represent value for money.

—   Rapidly rising costs for periodontal care are not consistent with the evidence of lower levels of advanced periodontal disease in the population and the concept that preventive maintenance should result in savings.

In response to the problems in financing periodontal care, private insurers in Ontario are modifying plans to:

—   Cover scaling only when done by a specialist.
—   Cover only 50% of costs compared with 80-100% of costs now covered.
—   Reduce the annual allowance for scaling.

These all might have an impact of the access to care. He pointed out the need for dentists to search for ways to address these concerns to ensure that dental insurance can continue.

Using data from an ongoing study of dental needs and care for adults in Ontario, James Leak demonstrated that among older dental patients in the Toronto, North York, Simcoe and Sudbury areas of Ontario, university level of education, visiting regularly for check-ups and living in Toronto, North York or Simcoe were the significant determinants of getting periodontal care. Neither insurance nor need factors (as reported by the subjects) were significant determinants.

James Beck raised the issue of the switch in orientation occurring in the U.S.A. to outcomes rather than services, i.e., plan sponsors want to pay only for procedures which are needed and which have benefit. Cost increases in health care in the United States are a real problem and cost containment has been an utter failure (cost-cutters cost more than money saved). He stated that society cannot provide everything to everyone as the means to deliver a service to those who would benefit. He feels that we need to develop predictor models of who is at most risk (to lose function or attachment) and have better evidence of therapies which reduce their risk. There is a danger in promising too much too soon and, therefore, much work needs to be done before we can implement such a scheme. However, this approach is in the mutual interest of the profession and insurers.

Summary

The group reported several broad conclusions for consideration:

—   Access to periodontal care is a problem for older adults.

—   While income may not be a predictor among patients, it is a predictor of access to regular care.

—   It seems morally repugnant to ask dentists to pay for the care of seniors by reducing their fees. (For example, Society doesn't ask gerontologists to subsidize the medical care for the elderly nor asks teachers of courses such as English as a Second Language to work for less because their clients are special).

—   We should end the artificial separation of nonpayment for periodontal infections compared with other infections in our provincial (or state) health care programs.

—   There are funds available to divert to such support. Members pointed to the monies inefficiently applied to supporting drug benefits for the elderly or to the universal provision of topical fluorides in fluoridated cities such as Toronto.

—   There are more issues than these which we need to explore through relevant research and conferences such as this.

Chapter 12
Maximizing Access to Periodontal Care:
Periodontal Health Promotion

H. Asuman Kiyak, Patricia M. Johnson, Daniel Kandelman, and David Locker

In an attempt to assure that all panelists and audience members could approach this topic from a similar perspective, the panel proposed three objectives for this workshop. These objectives were adapted for periodontal care from the broader report on health promotion from the Department of Health and Welfare Canada, *Achieving Health for All: A Framework for Health Promotion*.[1] The objectives that were addressed in varying ways by panel members were:

1. To reduce inequities in oral health status among subgroups of older populations.
2. To promote oral health as part of total health.
3. To provide comprehensive oral disease prevention programs that include a focus on periodontal health, and to make them culturally and linguistically relevant to diverse groups of elderly.

In the Canadian report cited above, these three objectives are described as "challenges" that are aimed especially at high risk groups. Unfortunately, in the area of oral health, many subgroups of elderly (ethnic and racial minorities, older women, those with inadequate retirement income) may be described as being at high risk for oral diseases. To the extent that the objectives or challenges described above can be met, we can expect gradual improvements in the quality of life for these high risk adults. The remainder of this workshop revolved around the efforts by panelists, members of the audience, and other programs known to the group on methods of achieving the oral health objectives described above. In particular, Dr. Jack Lee, Director of Dental Services for the City of Toronto, who participated in this panel, had chaired a committee on oral health promotion which was formed in 1988 by Health and Welfare Canada. Many of the recommendations of that committee, reported in Oral Health in Canada,[2] are consistent with those of this panel. Because health promotion plays a key role in achieving these objectives and is even part of this workshop title, it is useful to provide a working definition of health promotion, again derived from *Achieving Health for All*:

> *Health promotion* = The process of enabling people to enhance their control over and to improve their own health. It is the process of *empowerment*, and can be achieved through improved knowledge about self-care (e.g., health education programs aimed

at elderly themselves), mutual aid between elders and their peers, or with health providers (e.g., inservice training, caregiver manuals), and through the establishment of healthy environments (e.g., eliminating water and air pollution, adding fluoride to community water supplies).

A framework for achieving these objectives through a multi-faceted health promotion effort was introduced from the Canadian Report,[1] and is presented in Figure 1. *Panelists and audience members* discussed the feasibility of this framework for oral health promotion, especially in the area of periodontal health maintenance.

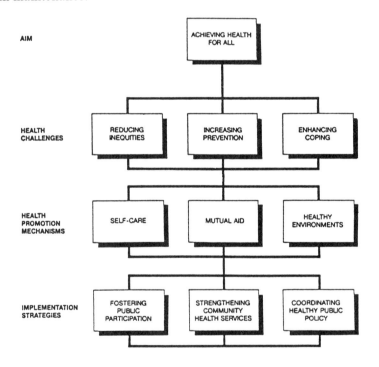

*From: Achieving Health for All: A Framework for Health Promotion.
       Ottawa: Department of Health and Welfare Canada, 1986, p.8.

Figure 1

As Figure 1 illustrates, it is important to foster public participation in health promotion efforts. In the case of periodontal health care, this includes involving older adults and their communities in the development of oral health education and delivery systems. Examples of this include public health programs with elderly members as board members to establish policies and methods of delivering dental care to their isolated and/or frail peers, or health education programs with elders who serve as educators or peer counsellors, together with a dental professional who provides the major content to be taught, but relies on an elder "co-educator" to disseminate the information in a manner that other elders in a given setting will most readily accept. Such collaboration between elders and dental providers is crucial, and in fact must be expanded to include organizations that promote the well-being of older adults (e.g., the American Association of Retired Persons) and dental product manufacturers that stand to profit from greater oral health awareness among older consumers.

This latter group can be especially effective in reaching the isolated elder through mass media. Television in particular may serve as the sole source of education and information for isolated, homebound elders and those with linguistic and cultural differences that preclude their active participation in senior centres and other venues for interaction with other elders. Indeed, television can be an important tool for educating elders, even those who do participate in community activities, since the older population generally spends more hours watching TV than other age groups.[3] Unfortunately, however, most dental product manufacturers have done little to educate elderly consumers about improving their oral health. For example, commercials for denture adhesives leave the viewer with the impression that poorly-fitting dentures are a necessary evil, and that their particular brand of adhesive will solve the problem! No mention is made of the fact that denture fit can change as the aging oral-facial structures change shape, or that elders should seek professional dental care for this problem. The implicit message of much of the dental product advertising is that young people have teeth and the elderly wear dentures! Rarely is an elderly person shown using a whitening toothpaste or mouthwash; these products are used by younger actors in TV commercials, resulting in a subliminal message that physical attractiveness, sex appeal, and social acceptance in general are the domain of the young.

Ad campaigns for dental product manufacturers reflect an awareness of what younger people seek in dental products—i.e., how to achieve whiter, straighter, more attractive teeth and a more attractive smile, and to avoid bad breath. These objectives may also be important for older audiences, but the advertising experts have rarely explored these issues, for whatever reasons. In fact, in an ongoing study of older adults from diverse cultures in Toronto and Seattle, it is surprising that these diverse elders have concurred on three major goals of oral health for themselves: maintaining their ability to chew a wide variety of foods, retaining as many teeth as possible, *and looking attractive*[4]. Surely the dental product advertisers can capitalize on these goals of older adults in their advertising for toothpaste, mouthwash or antibacterial rinses!

PROGRAM PLANNING KIT

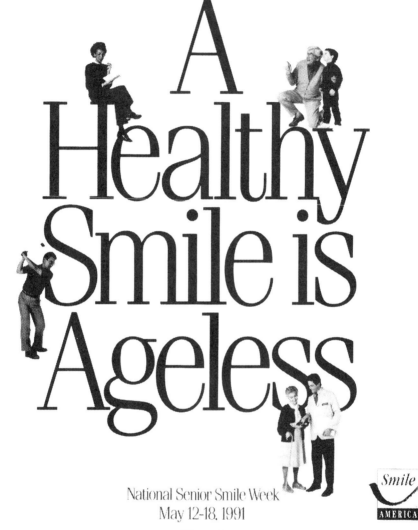

National Senior Smile Week
May 12-18, 1991

Figure 2
Copyright by the American Dental Association. Reprinted by permission.

Public participation in health promotion efforts can also take the form of community-wide oral health education campaigns for elders (e.g., "National

Senior Smile Week" is a campaign sponsored by the American Dental Association in May of every year in the United States; see Figure 2 for sample poster), free oral health screenings by local dental and hygienist organizations in senior centres, nursing homes and other settings where elderly congregate, and education programs for caregivers of frail elderly. A successful example of the latter is a recently completed program by Saxe and colleagues in Kentucky, Tennessee and West Virginia to educate home health care providers and family caregivers of elderly victims of stroke and Alzheimer's disease.[5] This program offered 3-4 hour workshops on oral health maintenance for caregivers of frail elderly in community settings, working in conjunction with home health agencies and support groups for families with victims of stroke and Alzheimer's disease.

Another implementation strategy for oral health promotion for elders is to strengthen community health services, not just dental, but general medical and social service programs, so that oral health efforts are coordinated with other services that might be more accessible to the elderly. The program in Kentucky, Tennessee and West Virginia, described above, used this strategy by collaborating with home health agencies (which traditionally have had easier access to homebound elders) and with caregiver support groups (who may be too overwhelmed by the physical and psychological burdens of caregiving to seek out dental care for their care recipients unless oral problems become acute).

The Ontario Oral Health Study,[6] reported by Dr. David Locker, highlighted this need for better coordination of dental services with other health programs, even for relatively independent elderly. In this survey of 907 elders, 60% had limitations in their activities of daily living (ADL) and 86% needed some oral hygiene instruction and/or care. It may be more feasible for other health care professionals to refer these people to dental services, or even to provide an initial oral health screening to these elders. This approach may result in greater utilization of dental services by older persons because the association between oral health and systemic health is implied if oral health screenings and educational messages are linked to general medical screenings.

A survey of homebound elderly in Quebec provided further support for the need to link oral health care with general medical care. In this survey of homebound elders, Dr. Daniel Kandelman and colleagues found that periodontal disease and denture problems, and the need for periodontal and denture care were more prevalent than in nursing home populations.[7] The role of TV in educating this population about oral health care was emphasized by Dr. Kandelman, who also suggested that the best dental care system for homebound elderly is through mobile dental visits. Hygienists should serve as the key dental professionals in mobile dental services since the majority of care is prevention (i.e., oral hygiene instruction, scaling, curettage). Hygienists could also serve a critical function in educating caregivers of homebound elderly, as well as nurses and nurse aides in long-term care facilities on oral health maintenance and in developing oral care plans for individual elderly. This would parallel the general care plan developed for each patient in long-term care facilities.

Panel members also emphasized the need to avoid stereotyping *all* elderly as high risk dental patients. Indeed, the regional surveys of Canadian elderly in Ontario and Quebec and of U.S. elderly in the National Adult Dental Survey,[8] have revealed significant differences across age cohorts. For example, the survey of elderly in Quebec found an average of 12 teeth per person in the young-old (ages 65-75); the rates in the U.S. survey were even higher. In contrast, the majority of the oldest-old (ages 85+) are edentulous. These two cohorts clearly have widely differing dental problems and needs. The need to distinguish *functional age* from *chronological age* in determining appropriate modes of dental care delivery was a significant conclusion of this panel.

Recommendations

Through the active participation of all panelists and audience members, the group developed a list of nine problem areas and recommendations to maximize access to periodontal care for the elderly. This report concludes with these recommendations:

1. It is important to attract qualified and dedicated dentists and hygienists into geriatric dentistry. The reality of lower potential earnings in this field, when compared with private practices where patients are primarily working adults with dental insurance, conflicts with a major motivation of many people who seek careers in dentistry or dental hygiene, i.e., high income and independent working conditions. This suggests the need to attract applicants with an interest in public health dentistry and special populations, even at the stage of entering DDS and RDH programs.

2. Perceived needs for older patients' dental care by providers may conflict with the perceptions of elders themselves. Furthermore, perceptions of other health care providers may conflict with objective assessments by dental professionals. These differences may be resolved by having dentists educate other health providers in long-term care facilities, and by working with these other health professionals to determine a realistic dental care plan for frail elderly.

3. Curricula in medicine and nursing need to include more on oral diseases and oral health maintenance than what is currently available.

4. While the medical and nursing professions need to learn more about oral diseases and oral health care, dentists must recognize that geriatric patients in long term care settings have complex and often frustrating health problems such that nurses and physicians who work in these settings must place many non-dental concerns higher in priority levels than oral health. This suggests the need for more research on the effects of oral conditions on systemic health. Otherwise non-dental professionals will continue to view oral health as a nice but not critical component of the older patient's overall well-being.

5. The survey of oral health in homebound elderly by Kandelman and colleagues[7] provides some insight into this neglected segment of the aged population. More surveys throughout North America are needed to provide further support for the significant oral health needs of these elderly. Along these lines, research is needed to ascertain the oral health needs of other high risk elderly.

6. Curricula of dental and dental hygiene programs often emphasize training in the technical aspects of dentistry rather than focusing on the goal of producing *oral health professionals*. This often results in a technically competent but unidimensional dentist or hygienist who has difficulty integrating the oral problems of patients with their medical, social, psychological, and economic status. This problem is underscored when dealing with frail elderly patients whose devastating oral conditions are merely part of a complex array of medical, social, psychological and economic problems.

7. Dental product manufacturers must be encouraged to work with experts in geriatric dentistry and to conduct focus groups with diverse elderly and their caregivers, in order to develop more appropriate advertising campaigns that not only sell products that fulfil older people's needs vis-à-vis oral health, but that also educate the elderly about oral health care in old age.

8. Public policy related to geriatric dental care must be changed; financial incentives must be offered in order to attract more dentists and hygienists into this field. These include the development of third party payment plans for dental care. Along these lines, legal regulations on dental practice must be addressed, including the opportunity for hygienists to do independent practice in community health care settings.

9. Finally, this panel asked a question which will require more systematic investigation by a broader cross-section of dentists, health care providers, policy makers and gerontologists: Can we afford "ideal" dental care for all citizens? Given that the Canadian report that started this discussion was entitled *Achieving Health for All*, it is reasonable to ask if this is a reasonable goal in oral health care. Perhaps a more appropriate question is "What is the minimal level of oral health that all elderly should have a right to expect?" Only when this question has been addressed satisfactorily can we expect to maximize access to periodontal and other oral health care for the elderly.

Endnotes

1. *Department of Health and Welfare Canada.* Achieving Health for All: A Framework for Health Promotion. Ottawa: Minister of Supply and Services, 1986.

2. Health and Welfare Canada. Final Report of oral health promotion committee. *Oral Health in Canada: Facing the Future* (Chair: Dr. Jack Lee), 1991.

3. Gordon, D., Gaitz, CM. & Scott, J. Leisure and lives: Personal expressivity across the lifespan. In R. Binstock and E. Shanas (Eds), *Handbook of Aging and the Social Sciences*, New York: Van Nostrand, 1976.

4. This survey of elderly users of Toronto Public Health Department dental services and Seattle senior centre members is a collaborative effort of Drs. Jack Lee and Bruce Schaef of Toronto, and Dr. Asuman Kiyak of the University of Washington, Seattle.

5. Saxe, S., Henry, RG., Wekstein, MW., Brooks, JD., Meckstroth, RL. & Smith, TA. Final Report: Oral Health Care Strategies for Family Caregivers of Dependent Homebound Elderly in Appalachia. *University of Kentucky.* AOA Grant No. 90AT0336, 1991.

6. Locker, D., Leake, J. & Otchere, D. Study of Oral Health and Treatment Needs of Ontario's Current and Future Elderly. *Department of Community Dentistry. University of Toronto.* 1991.

7. Kandelman, D. Survey of Housebound Elderly in Quebec, Canada. Unpublished, 1991.

8. NIDR. Oral Health of United States Adults: National Findings. DHHS:NIDR, *NIH Publication* No. 87-2868, 1987.

Chapter 13
Managing and Motivating the Oral Hygiene Needs of Independently Living Older Adults

Margery G.E. Forgay, Sharon M. Aitken, Pierre Baehni and Nils Ravald

Introduction

Demographic shifts in Western countries are resulting in an increased proportion of seniors in the population. This has resulted in an increased focus on the health-related needs of older adults. The major focus has been on needs of the institutionalized elderly, but in reality, most seniors live independently, and therefore require different approaches to the prevention of disease and maintenance of health. In particular, this group must be assisted in managing their own health maintenance as much as possible.

Identifying Needs, Resources, and Barriers

Needs and Resources

American and Scandinavian studies have shown that elderly people are gradually retaining more teeth.[1,2] The prevalence of natural teeth seems to be related to a number of factors, including socioeconomic status, lifestyle, and chronological age.[3-6] Moreover, the general improvement of health, improved medical and dental care and higher demands from the social environment make people more aware of the importance of good oral health conditions.

There is little evidence that we have improved oral health through better dietary habits. Thus, the explanation for the improvement must be found elsewhere. The importance of fluoride administration has been clearly demonstrated in communities with different fluoride contents in the water.[7,8] The use of fluoride-containing tooth-pastes[1] has undoubtedly been of crucial importance in the reduction of caries. The epidemiological study by Hugoson et al.[2] showed improved oral hygiene in all age-groups. Also, a positive correlation has been shown between the frequency of toothbrushing and remaining teeth.[9] Moreover, people in all age-groups use toothbrushes and interdental cleaning aids such as dental floss and toothpicks on a regular basis more than before.[10]

Long-term improvements not only in caries rates but in periodontal health have been demonstrated. The improvement in periodontal health is not so evident in the elderly as in the overall population, due to more retained teeth and accumulated periodontal lesions over time.[11,12] However, at least in the

Scandinavian countries, improved oral hygiene and dental care have significantly altered the pattern of periodontal disease in all age-groups.[2]

Although the general tendency to better oral health is obvious, there are individuals or groups of individuals at greater risk for dental disorders. A relatively higher proportion of these individuals is found in the older age-groups. This is due to impaired general health, medication and changes in social circumstances rather than to aging *per se*.

What is the general health of older adults? In a Swedish study in Gothenburg it has been shown that most people aged above 70 years of age are in good physical and mental condition.[13] In fact, a higher mental capacity in older age-groups than before has been demonstrated. However, large individual differences exist. The difference is accentuated with age. Therefore, it is not meaningful to discuss chronological age in the elderly, but rather biological age.

The proportion of older adults who are institutionalized in Western countries varies, but in all cases is low. From the Gothenburg studies, we know that only 3% of 70-year-old people are institutionalized. At age of 79, 90% live independently at their homes. Only 2% of the 70-year-olds, 4% of the 75-year-olds and 9% of 79-year-old people have severe handicaps. This is somewhat in contrast with reports from the U.S.A., where as may as 40% of the older population have been reported to have special needs based on complex health problems and functional status.[14]

Most older adults live in their own homes. It can be concluded that most individuals living independently are in good enough physical and mental condition to be capable of receiving dental health information and hopefully acting according to instructions. How well we succeed depends to a great extent upon how our message is presented. As pointed out by Gift,[15] this may require "special attention to methods of communication, including message structuring, repetition and reinforcement, shorter session length, information limitations, active participation and multiple modes of presentation".

Most elderly adults continue to live in their own homes. We may also suppose that people who have been seeking dental services will also in the future. Although incomes may be less, individuals may have more time to spend on health promotion, including oral hygiene. For this group, general information about caries, especially root caries, and periodontal disease should be provided, in combination with an individually designed recall program.

Barriers
In the groups of elderly adults that only now occasionally seek dental services, the chief problem is that their perceived oral health status does not reflect the actual clinical situation. It has been shown that the older the patient and the

fewer teeth present, the lower is the subjective demand for dental service.[16] Other barriers to oral hygiene and treatment are such factors as financial barriers, lack of dental hygiene and treatment traditions, cultural differences, lack of knowledge about where or how to get treatment, edentulousness, general illness and handicaps, fear of dental treatment, transportation difficulties and negative attitudes to dental care and treatment (from relatives, children, husbands or wives). If we want to be successful, these factors must be considered.

In an attempt to overcome some of the above-mentioned barriers, a project was performed in the Swedish county of Dalarna.[17] All inhabitants 65 years and older (54,000 individuals), were offered, by personal letter, a free dental examination if they were without dental care. Eighty-eight per cent of the population answered. Of those responding, 47% answered that they were without regular dental care. Almost 50% of these wanted to get a dental examination. Thus, 10,000 new patients were identified and treated individually. This project was performed by the Public Dental Health Service, and both public dental surgeons and private dental clinics all over the county participated. Thereby, the travel for each individual was minimized. The cost for the project (excluding treatment costs) was calculated to be about $20 U.S. per individual attending examination. It was thus shown that dental services can be offered at a low cost with a good response by individuals with an earlier low attendance for dental care.

Potential Results

What results could we expect of our hygiene procedures in the elderly? Are seniors capable of maintaining oral hygiene at a high level after treatment? Behavioural research suggests that attitudes and knowledge of oral health can be modified even in older subjects.[20] Indeed studies have shown that oral hygiene can be improved through behavioural approach and self-monitoring techniques. This approach aims not only at increasing the individual's awareness and responsibility for oral health but also attempts to enhance self-esteem and psychological well-being.

Most studies in this field show temporary changes in attitudes following educational programs on health promotion but fail to demonstrate any long-term effect. However, the possibilities of improving and maintaining dental hygiene at a good level have been shown in short-term[18] and long-term[19] clinical trials. In a study by Knazan,[18] the possibilities of improving oral hygiene and gingival health by using a diagnostic approach to health education were demonstrated. Axelsson et al.[19] recently reported results from a 15-year follow-up of patients maintained on a high standard of oral hygiene. During the last

9 years, 95% of the patients only visited dental hygienists once or twice a year. At the baseline examination, the individuals between 51 and 70 years showed a mean plaque score of 60%. At the 15-year follow-up, the plaque score was 15%. The overall caries incidence was extremely low. Almost all carious lesions were secondary to old fillings or restorations. The probing pocket depths and clinical attachment levels were maintained or improved throughout the observation period. Thus, if we can get the patients to maintain good oral hygiene standards and attend follow-ups by dental hygienists, dental caries and periodontal disease in older adults can be prevented. There is a need for more long-term studies on specific behavioural interventions and their affects on periodontal health.

Oral Health Promotion and Disease Prevention

There is a demonstrated lack of dental awareness among the present group of older individuals.[16] Oral health is perceived to be less important than general physical health. Regular professional dental care is not sought by many older subjects. In the over 65 age group approximately 35 to 42% are edentulous. Only about 30 to 40% have visited a dentist during the preceding year, with a much lower rate in the edentulous group. Pain and emergency situations are the most common reasons for the most recent dental visit. Many factors may explain this low priority given to oral health by older persons. Lack of perceived need is one of the major reasons for not seeking dental care, especially among edentulous persons. Present-day older people seem to be resigned to accepting their oral health condition and most believe that they will eventually lose their teeth. Yet they express, in general, positive attitudes toward prevention and oral health. Oral hygiene is often neglected and plaque retention represents a major problem. Decreased oral cleanliness may be due to plaque retention because of iatrogenic restorations, root surface caries or root exposure as a consequence of periodontal disease, as well as diminished manual dexterity or loss of motivation. However, it is interesting to note that for most older adults with natural teeth, brushing is considered the most important preventive measure to maintain oral health. A significant proportion of dentate older individuals also report flossing on a regular basis. The overall picture is not as grim as it looks. Significant improvement in oral health status, changes in attitude toward oral health, as well as in utilization patterns of dental services have been observed over these past decades.

Promotion of oral health and prevention is a multifaceted problem.[15] Prevention practices, regardless of age, include self-care and professional care. Self-care consists of adequate plaque control by toothbrushing with fluoride toothpaste, interdental as well as denture cleaning, use of fluoride rinse, regular visits to the dentist, and adequate dietary habits. Attitudes toward oral health and capacity for self-care depend on a multitude of variables and experiences accumulated over a lifetime.

Consider some key questions concerning oral health promotion among independent older subjects. Who should receive dental services? Instead of aiming at all groups without distinction, oral health promotion and prevention should be targeted and tailored to meet the specific needs of groups of individuals. As stated earlier, elderly people represent a very heterogeneous population. Groups such as the institutionalized and handicapped can be readily identified and have the poorest oral health among the elderly.

In addition, recent epidemiological research has shown that certain groups of people are more at risk to develop dental caries and periodontal diseases. Identification of older adults who are at risk for periodontal disease will require the development of some methods to identify and assess risk influences. Advances in diagnostic technology using microbiological, biological and genetic markers will help. For example, levels of mutans streptococci above 10^6 mL of saliva in young individuals is a good predictor of a person at risk to develop caries. Tests are currently becoming available for detecting the presence of periodontal pathogens. Such tests will help to identify individuals or groups of subjects who are at risk and need active preventive cares. These tests will also be useful to monitor the efficacy of our preventive measures and consequently in patient management. One example of a test already frequently used by patients at home is the use of dental plaque disclosing agents. Another possibility for patients to check their gingival conditions is to perform gingival bleeding tests.[21,22] Such tests might in the future be used by medical and dental allied health personnel, or by patients themselves, to determine the level of hygiene needed to maintain oral health. One perplexing problem at present is what plaque levels individuals can tolerate and still maintain oral health.

To identify medical and dental risk groups, the dental profession should cooperate more closely with medical and social professionals. As many as 120 physical or mental disorders may cause symptoms in the oral cavity or affect the patient's ability to perform dentally related tasks.[15] The prevalence of most of these conditions increases with increased age. We meet patients of this type in their homes and at institutions. Their dental problems are often of minor importance compared with their general health problems, but severely diseased people often need help with oral hygiene measures. The problem might not be to identify, but rather to motivate these patients and their helpers to provide dental hygiene.

What types of preventive methods should be applied? During the past decade there has been a noticeable shift from treatment of disease to prevention, especially in younger age groups. Efforts to promote oral health should now be pursued with older populations. Use of behavioural interventions to improve oral health perception and compliance with dental care regimens may hold some promises and should be encouraged. One should also note that changes in attitudes and preventive practices may gradually change as upcoming cohorts will have better oral health and will be more knowledgeable and more prevention-oriented. Another way to improve oral health perception could be through mass media, nondental organizations, and industry. They have the potential to deliver messages targeted to older individuals but their role has not been fully explored.

Some questions will still need to be addressed concerning the efficacy of specific preventive interventions. It will be essential, for example, to clarify whether the preventive measures that are effective in children are as equally effective with older adults. As oral hygiene remains a pivotal component of prevention, the appropriate level of plaque control to be attained should be determined. In the future, we could anticipate changes in the type of preventive measures and methods applied. Development of new biomaterials and new delivery methods of pharmacologically active agents will certainly play an important role in prevention in elderly populations.[24] Preventive coatings for the protection of all exposed tooth surfaces, composite resins, varnishes as well as sustained release devices or local delivery systems will be developed. Research in the field of biomaterials is very promising and in some instances these new materials are already available. These new delivery systems will be able to release fluoride, antimicrobial agents or saliva-stimulating agents directly in the mouth for prolonged periods of time. These developments should provide powerful preventive tools especially important for individuals at risk or people who are physically or mentally handicapped.

Canada's Baby Boomers as Older Adults

Canada's aging population presents some interesting challenges for both health care institutions and health care professionals. Major changes in Canadian life have often been defined in terms of how the "baby boom" generation moves in and out of its various growth phases. The retirement/geriatric phase is likely to place the greatest strain yet on the social fabric of the Canadian mosaic.

Having funded most of the new initiatives in the government's growing social contract, baby boomers will rightfully expect a high level of support as they reach their own retirement phase; yet this largest single identifiable generation will enter old age at a time when this social contract between the government and its citizens is under the greatest strain. The safety net of Canadian social programs will not likely be reliable. Current thinking already predicts that the Canada Pension Plan will be hard pressed to meets its obligations. Demographically speaking, the tax base will be too small to support the pensionable population.

Following a lifetime of increased focus on personal health issues (ie., diet, exercise, weight loss, personal appearance, nonsmoking) baby boomers will enter the fixed income phase of their lives with a history of access to universal medical care and third-party dental insurance. Presumably healthier and with most of their teeth, they will be motivated to continue accessing regular dental care, while living on lower than expected fixed incomes, and without dental care being funded by previous employers.

Managing Oral Hygiene Needs: A Need for a Change

How will this generation of seniors manage their oral hygiene needs? We can anticipate a vocal demand for access to low cost no-frills maintenance procedures. We should also anticipate an extensive reliance on home health care maintenance, perhaps in the form of simple diagnostic tests and home do-it-yourself aids. What can the dental and allied dental professions do to meet the needs of these healthy, yet not always so wealthy, independent, older adults?

Clearly, the dental profession cannot assume that the use of dental services by the elderly will continue to increase as a function of preventive efforts. The dental profession will have to undergo a significant shift in its attitudes to meet the expectations of this generation. Quite apart from its relationship with health professions, this generation has had to develop an entirely new response to the pressures of making a living in a competitive international marketplace. Although protected by professional bodies from international competition, health professions need to recognize that their patients are developing international standards of customer service against which they will measure professional services. The temptation to dismiss these trends as short-term fads should be resisted. Health professions need to appreciate that the trends represent a fundamental change in the economic competitiveness of the Western world. The impact has been no less than a major upheaval in the traditional relationship between customers and suppliers. There is no reason to believe that the relationship between professionals and their clients will escape the same pressures.

Baby boomers are increasingly vocal. Once the silent majority, they have rejected the acquiescent role of society's provider, and are now more likely to demand their due. They demand of others what has been demanded of them: Total Quality Management (TQM) of whatever service they receive: that is, the best possible product and the best possible price, at the best level of service. Having been forced to rethink their own attitudes in order to survive, they are unlikely to have any sympathy for those who have not kept pace. Their demands on the health care system will not be placated by excuses of systemic ineffectiveness. Although some will be able to elect for unique treatment plans, the majority can be expected to demand basic care and maintenance at increasingly competitive prices. Innovative approaches will be demanded at every turn.

Options for Future Directions

Funding
As many individuals indicate that cost of care is not a barrier for use of dental service,[15,17,18] the financial barriers may seem to be somewhat overestimated. However, real poverty must be considered. Each country has its own system(s) of dental insurance. Regardless of the system, general basic dental service should be offered to the elderly population, i.e., basic relief from pain, an acceptable function of the dentition and the possibility of keeping the dentition in health by oral hygiene measures. Unfortunately, the public dental health expenditures in the Western countries are decreasing, thereby making it more difficult to meet the dental costs for the elderly. Government programs must become more efficient and cost effective so that they can provide a higher level of care to a greater number of people. In the short term, more and more dental insurance plans will need to include an option which allows participants to pay now for regular maintenance dental care after retirement. As a "Sunset Option", it will provide for regular care while seniors are in the fixed income phase of their lives.

Retirement Information and Planning
Presently, retirement information and planning programs tend to focus on paying off the mortgage and owning a car free and clear. Why couldn't they also include a section on the importance of getting one's mouth in a state of good repair, while they are still covered by dental insurance and before they are medically compromised? The mouth is the first area of the body to be neglected amongst people who suffer from chronic illness.[25] Elimination of areas of plaque retention on tooth surfaces and restorations by replacing old or poorly fitting restorations would make the mouth more self-cleansing and easier for the patient to maintain.

Lifestyle and Health Education Programs
Health information and education programs should include more information on the importance of teeth. They should emphasize the fact that potential nutritional and health problems often result from a limited or non-existent chewing capacity and that teeth contribute to a person's mental health by providing a sense of well-being associated with appearance and speech.

Private Dental Practice
Periodontal care for most older adults will be provided by dentists and dental hygienists in general dental practice settings. Only a small proportion will be treated by periodontists. There is an urgent need to expand and improve the education of undergraduate dental and allied dental personnel in a wide spectrum of issues on aging as well as in provision of dental care.

The dental profession must also address the idiosyncrasy of practising in isolation, away from the mainstream of the health care system. Older people are more likely than any other age group to use physician and other health services.[20] Therefore, dental care for seniors, whether privately or publicly funded, must be provided in multi-disciplinary/interdisciplinary service centres. The dental profession must communicate more with physicians and other allied health professions to educate them in the recognition of active or potential dental problems. Effort should especially be made to heighten awareness of these professions about dental matters and oral health promotion for elderly patients.

With a shift to health maintenance care and treatment in the community, privately practising dentists, hygienists and technicians could extend their services beyond the scope of their stationary physical facilities to senior citizens at community centres, community health clinics, or seniors centres. This could be accomplished through the use of mobile units or portable equipment. Such shared equipment could be operated by individual entrepreneurs, coordinated effort by local dental societies or even the government.

Other Options Include:
— Diagnostic services to recognize early dysfunction or disease by identifying high-risk patients. The use of a simple diagnostic tools for testing biological parameters, such as collagenase and gelatinase assays in mouthrinse samples (currently being researched at the University of Toronto) could be used to identify persons with periodontitis.[26] Similarly, there are many such avenues currently being pursued in research or being reviewed by regulatory bodies of governments.

— The use of fluoride and antimicrobial rinses as an adjunct to home oral hygiene care.

— The mass media are most effective in reaching older adults; focusing health promotion messages through these channels.

— Educational services to improve prevention and instruction to seniors.

— In conjunction with such agencies such as Seniors For Seniors, or Senior Peer Helping Programs, a coordinated monitoring service to ensure that appropriate dental health actions are undertaken by the seniors themselves.

— Coordination of publicly financed programs with personal resources and identifying supplemental support for dental services from a multitude of philanthropic and community organizations.

— Improved education of undergraduate dental and dental hygiene students.

Providers of Oral Health Care

A final question may be, "Is it always necessary to use personnel from the dental professions to identify oral hygiene needs?" The potential role of nonhealth professionals or even lay-people should also be explored. Indeed, such "oral health educators" already exist in different countries such as Sweden and Switzerland. Such new types of auxiliaries may prove to be extremely cost-efficient and rewarding on a human and emotional level for both the care giver and the patient.

Dental public health programs must be based on a multidisciplinary model for monitoring and assessing dental care needs. Dental personnel must broaden their responsibilities by educating, motivating, frequently evaluating and providing feedback to para and allied health professions (e.g., visiting nurses, social workers, mental health workers, counsellors). This is particularly important in the case of reaching the not-so-healthy independently living seniors. These older adults will rely extensively on home visiting allied health professions to provide monitoring and assessment of dental care needs as well as other needs.

We can increase manpower by using volunteers with seniors to conduct follow-up (monitoring) and provide additional reinforcement in dental health care.

Another way to be more cost efficient is for dental personnel to identify other care givers in the community, such as relatives and neighbours, and provide them with a support mechanism to help maintain the dental hygiene need of seniors.

No matter which approach is used to manage the dental hygiene needs of independently living seniors, the process must be humanized. Elderly persons require special attention, skills, and understanding. The dental professions need to adopt a more caring attitude and willingness to serve this population.

Conclusion

Health and autonomy are important issues for older adults.[27] The state of oral health in the later years of life depends on genetic, socioeconomic, behavioural, and environmental factors. New patterns of oral health status and attitudes, and new needs will be emerging as younger generations of adults will reach old age. Oral health promotion and prevention will therefore be affected by these changes. In addition, technical developments and changes in dental service organizations will occur and will help provide better care to the elderly.

Endnotes

1. Ismail AI, Burt BA, Hendershot GE, Jack S, Corbin SB. Findings from the dental care supplement of the National Health Interview Survey, 1983. *J Am Dent Assoc.* 1987;114:617-21.
2. Hugoson A, Kock G, Bergendal T et al. Oral health of individuals aged 3-80 years in Jönköping, Sweden, in 1973 and 1983. II. A review of clinical and radiographic findings. *Swed Dent J.* 1986;10:175-94.
3. Baum BJ. Characteristics of participants in the oral physiology component of the Baltimore Longitudinal Study of Aging. *Community Dent Oral Epidemiol.* 1981;9:128-34.
4. Österberg T, Mellström D. Tobacco smoking: a major risk factor for loss of teeth in three 70-year-old cohorts. *Community Dent Oral Epidemiol.* 1986;14:367-70.
5. Österberg T, Hedegård B, Säther G. Variation in dental health in 70-year-old men and women in Gothenburg, Sweden. A cross-sectional epidemiological study including longitudinal and cohort effects. *Swed Dent J.* 1983;7:29-48.
6. Palmkvist S, Österberg T, Mellström D. Oral health and socioeconomic factors in a Swedish county population aged 65 and over. *Geriodontics.* 1986;2:138-42.
7. Burt BA, Ismail AI, Eklund SA. Root caries in an optimally fluoridated and a high-fluoride community. *J Dent Res.* 1986;65:1154-8.
8. Brustman B. Impact of exposure to fluoride-adequate water on root surface caries in elderly. *Gerodontics.* 1986;2:203-7.
9. Vehkalahti M, Paunio I. Remaining teeth in Finnish adults related to the frequency of tooth-brushing. *Acta Odontol Scand.* 1989;47:375-381.
10. Uhrbom E, Bjerner B. EPIWUX 88. An epidemiological study of oral health in adults in the county of Dalarna, Sweden. A cross-sectional and longitudinal study 1983-1988 (in Swedish). *Department of Public Dental Health Service.* Falun, Sweden, 1988.
11. Douglass C, Gillings D, Sollecito W, Gammon M. The potential for increase in the periodontal disease of the aged population. *J Periodontol.* 1983;54:721-30.
12. Page R. Periodontal disease in the elderly: A critical evaluation of current information. *Gerodontology.* 1984;3:63-70.
13. Svanborg A. Seventy-year-old people in Gothenburg. A population study in an industrialized Swedish city. II. General presentation of social and medical conditions. *Acta Med Scand.* 1977;611:5-37.
14. Personnel for health needs of the elderly through the year 2000. Draft Report to Congress for the Secretary, *U.S. Department of Health and Human Services.* March 1987.

15.   Gift HC. Issues of aging and oral health promotion. *Gerodontics.* 1988;4:194-06.
16.   Rise J, Holst D. Causal analysis on the use of dental services among old-age pensioners in Norway. *Community Dent Oral Epidemiol.* 1982;10:167-72.
17.   Uhrbom E, Bjerner B. Dental care for elderly in W-county. A co-operation project between public and private dental clinics (in Swedish). *Department of Public Dental Health Service.* Falun, Sweden, 1987.
18.   Knazan YL. Application of PRECEDE to dental health promotion for a Canadian well-elderly population. *Gerodontics.* 1986;2:180-5.
19.   Axelsson P, Lindhe J, Nyström B. On the prevention of caries and periodontal disease. Results of a 15-year longitudinal study in adults. *J Clin Periodontol.* 1991;18:182-9.
20.   Kiyak HA. Recent advances in behavioural research in geriatric dentistry. *Gerodontology.* 7:27-36, 1988.
21.   Glavind L, Attström R. Periodontal self-examination, a motivation tool in periodontics. *J Clin Periodontol.* 1979;6:238-51.
22.   Kallio P, Ainamo J, Dusadeepan A. Self-assessment of gingival bleeding—ringbell for improved oral hygiene. *Int Dent J.* 1990;40:231-6.
23.   Ravald N, Hamp S-E, Birkhed D. Long-term evaluation of root surface caries in periodontally treated patients. *J Clin Periodontol.* 1986;13:758-67.
24.   Broadening the Scope. Long-range Research Plan for the Nineties. *National Institute of Dental Research.* NIH Publication No. 9-1188, 1990.
25.   Lebel JL. Health needs of the elderly. *Dental Clinics of North America.* 33(1):1-5, 1989.
26.   Gangbar S, McCulluch CAG, Overall CM, Sodek J. Identification of polymorphonuclear leukocyte collagenase and gelatinase activities in mouthrinse samples: Correlation with periodontal disease activity in adult and juvenile periodontitis. *J Periodont Res.* 1990;25:257-267.
27.   A research agenda on oral health in the elderly. National Institute on Aging, *National Institute of Dental Research.* Veterans Administration, 1986.

Chapter 14
Modifying Standard Preventive Approaches for the Functionally Dependent and Disabled Elderly

Jonathan Ship, David W. Banting, Tim Gould and Laura Dempster

Prior to the discussion group meeting, the panel identified three major issues relating to the modification of standard preventive approaches for the functionally dependent and disabled elderly. These issues were:

1. mechanical and chemical plaque control procedures for the functionally dependent and disabled elderly;
2. the role of care-givers in the oral care of the functionally dependent and disabled elderly, and
3. policies and programs of oral care for the functionally dependent and disabled elderly.

For each of these issues, the panel collectively identified a number of questions which needed to be addressed. The questions, as determined by the panel, are provided as Appendix A. In the group discussion, the three issues were briefly summarized and some background material was provided with respect to each of the issues. Throughout its deliberations, the discussion group defined the functionally dependent and disabled elderly as older adults who were institutionalized or homebound due to chronic disabilities such as multiple sclerosis, Parkinson's disease, Alzheimer's disease, etc.

I. Mechanical and Chemical Plaque Control Procedures for the Functionally Dependent and Disabled Elderly

Studies on a variety of medically compromised and disabled elderly populations indicate that their oral health is diminished. Patients with mental illness and dementia (Whittle et al., 1987), Parkinson's disease (Jolly et al., 1989), Alzheimer's disease (Ship, 1989; Ship et al., 1990), mental retardation (Thornton et al., 1989, Pieper et al., 1986; Sanger & Casamassimo, 1983), bipolar disorders (Friedlander & Birch, 1990), neuromuscular, seizure, and respiratory disorders (Sanger & Casamassimo, 1983) have impaired oral health. Therefore, it appears that there are special oral health needs by the functionally dependent and disabled elderly.

The data base on this subject is poor. Most research studying utilization patterns of dental services neglect information pertinent to the medical status of the participants. One paper by Gilbert et al. 1990) suggests that community dwelling, cognitively impaired elders are at risk for low use of dental care, which may have consequences for their oral health. Alternatively, traditional health care barriers such as sensory handicaps, poor general health, and infrequent physician barriers have been found to lack significance regarding dental and medical visits (Evashwick et al., 1984; Branch et al., 1986). It appears that the most accurate predictors of both medical and dental service use is perceived need, as experienced by the patient (Kiyak, 1987).

There are volumes of literature detailing mechanical and chemical plaque control procedures for community-dwelling healthy young individuals. Unfortunately, there are little data describing specific preventive measures for the elderly disabled. Chlorhexidine mouthrinses combined with supervised tooth brushing were shown to be effective in controlling plaque levels and gingivitis in young mentally retarded institutionalized patients (Brayer et al., 1985). Chlorhexidine rinse and spray as an adjunct to oral hygiene and gingival health in physically and mentally handicapped adults resulted in lower plaque and bleeding scores, and slightly diminished pocketing (Yanover et al, 1988; Kalaga et al., 1989). Data on healthy older subjects is also lacking, although a paper by Persson et al. (1991) found improved oral health in elderly subjects rinsing with chlorhexidine versus placebo controls. Abstracts from the 1991 International Association for Dental Research (IADR) meeting describe effective plaque control and diminished gingivitis with electric toothbrushes in hospital, nursing home, and retirement complex-dwelling elderly populations (Blahut et al., 1991; abstracts 801-803).

Researchers have attempted to find associations between manual dexterity and oral health, to see if improving manual dexterity skills would result in an improvement in oral hygiene. Positive correlations were found in "normal adults" between oral hygiene and manual dexterity (Kenney et al,, 1976), but not in handicapped adults (Shaw et al., 1989). Shaw et al. (1989) postulated that the periodontal status of their handicapped population was so poor, and the levels of comprehension and dexterity so low that any relationship which may have existed between the two was not demonstrable.

Many older persons suffer from salivary gland dysfunction and complain of xerostomia. This has been attributed to systemic disease and medication utilization, rather than aging itself (Ship & Baum, 1990). Functionally dependent and disabled older people are therefore susceptible to salivary gland dysfunction. Fortunately, there is a wealth of literature detailing the benefits of topical and systemic fluorides for the prevention of caries. For example, fluoridated dentifrices were shown to reduce the incidence of root and coronal caries in older adults (Jensen & Kohout, 1988), and residents in fluoridated communities had fewer caries and greater numbers of teeth compared to those in non-fluoridated communities (Hunt et al., 1989; Stamm et al., 1990). Since periodontal and gingival disease have been associated with cervical caries (e.g., DePaola et al., 1989; Kitamura et al., 1986; Locker et al., 1989), the maintenance of gingival and periodontal health in both healthy and compromised older adults should assist in the preservation of the natural dentition. Traditionally, these studies have been performed with community-dwelling persons or in carefully selected subjects for clinical trials. Little data exist on the relationship between periodontal health and dental caries in compromised older adults, and clinical trials should be instituted to examine the effects of fluoride versus placebo treatment in functionally dependent and disabled older individuals.

II. The Role of Care-Givers in Oral Care of the Functionally Dependent and Disabled Elderly

There has been much work devoted to oral hygiene practices of mentally retarded individuals and in the development of dental care programs for disabled patients. According to Nicolaci & Tesini (1982), oral hygiene can improve significantly, either by providing intensified daily brushing by dental personnel with the development of self-help workshops for residents, or by providing effective staff training. Some programs have emphasized the training of institutionalized direct-care staff (e.g., Nicolaci & Tesini, 1982; Wadsworth et al. 1986) and home-care staff (e.g., Davies & Whittle, 1990) in order to improve oral hygiene. An underlying theme in these programs for disabled adults is that greater oral hygiene supervision will result in diminished dental disease.

Providing dental care to disabled adults has also received attention in the literature. The consensus is that dental professionals should greatly emphasize preventive practices in these populations. Outpatient management of handicapped patients can be performed (Indresano & Rooney, 1981), and these patients can be treated in dental school clinics (Sigal et al., 1988), general dental practices (Davies et al., 1988), and in mobile dental programs with cost-effective strategies (Dane, 1990). Dental treatment planning for compromised patients should focus on patients' chief complaints and perceived needs, as well as medical, psychological, social, and economic factors which will influence treatment (Gordon & Sullivan, 1986). Finally, the hallmark of dental care for patients with life-long illnesses and declining function should be the preservation of function for as long a period of time as possible. Protocols describing these philosophies have been well documented for patients with dementia and Alzheimer's disease (Friedlander & Jarvik, 1987; Niessen et al., 1985; Niessen & Jones, 1986: Niessen & Jones, 1987a,b). With the increasing numbers of older persons in society and a concomitant increase in the numbers of disabled elderly, dental professionals should be trained to manage and treat these individuals.

III. Policies and Programs of Oral Care for the Functionally Dependent and Disabled Elderly

According to Public Law 100-230 in the United States, the Omnibus Reconciliation Act of 1987 (OBRA) has changed the requirements for dental care and services effective October 1, 1990. Patients In nursing homes covered under the U.S. Medicare system are to receive emergency and routine dental care as required. Medicaid patients must receive emergency dental care and routine dental care to the extent of the State Health Plan.

Regarding the effectiveness of institutional programs, several protocols have detailed the success of oral hygiene programs in a tertiary care setting (e.g., Nicolaci & Tesini, 1982; Wadsworth et al. 1986). There are scant data on patient and care-giver oral hygiene compliance. Henry et al. (1989) did find discrepancies between the reported frequency of administration of chlorhexidine mouth rinses as written per medical order in a hospital and its actual distribution as determined by the amount dispensed by trained nursing staff. Therefore, programs are necessary to train both patients and care-givers, but without adequate compliance, the overall effectiveness may be limited.

Conclusions and Recommendations

Preventive procedures
There was general agreement among the group participants that preventive procedures were not adequate for the functionally dependent and disabled elderly. However, it was acknowledged that, in many instances, the administration of preventive procedures to this population subgroup was limited both by technology and lack of compliance. It was also acknowledged that the functionally dependent and disabled elderly did not normally exhibit extensive periodontal problems involving irreversible disease. Rather, the issue was one of maintenance of oral hygiene rather than the provision of definitive and aggressive periodontal treatment.

Problems
The discussion group identified a number of problems which had an effect on the provision of standard preventive procedures to the functionally dependent and disabled elderly. These problems can be listed as follows:

1.   Attitudes Concerning Dental Health
Generally speaking, dental health is not viewed as having a high priority by other health professionals or by those providing nursing care (nursing staff and family) to the functionally dependent and disabled elderly. Furthermore, it was noted that the dental profession does not assert itself sufficiently in indicating to the other health professions and care-givers that it is responsible for a major organ system. The dental profession does not advocate the importance or the necessity of improved oral health care as much as it should.

2.   Physical and Mental Health of Patients
It was acknowledged that this type of patient is difficult to manage because of physical and mental disabilities and, therefore, the standard preventative approaches may need to be modified. An ideal outcome may not be a realistic expectation.

Utilization of, or demand for, dental services for the functionally dependent and disabled elderly probably reflects the perceived need as viewed by the patient's family. This was acknowledged to be generally low and it was felt that there was a need to improve the public's knowledge regarding the benefits and consequences of preventive dental care. Particularly, issues such as quality of life, improved self-image, focal infection, the risk of aspiration pneumonia and the effect of the dentition on food selection were mentioned.

Solutions
The discussion group identified many areas that needed improvement but focused on those areas that would most likely result in an improvement in the oral care of the functionally dependent and disabled elderly. These were as follows:

1.   Education
It was felt that there was an immediate need to educate care-givers, institution administrators, the family, the general public, the dental profession and other health professions with respect to the importance of oral care for the functionally dependent and disabled elderly. This might be accomplished through both formal programs such as the RNA programs at the Community College level or, more informally, community outreach types of activities. In hospitals it can be provided directly via hospital dental staff personnel.

2.   Initiation of Oral Care Programs within Institutions
It was agreed that formal programs of mouth-care should be introduced at institutions caring for the functionally dependent and disabled elderly. However, by necessity, the programs will vary widely depending on the local situation.

Nevertheless, there are some basic standards or principles which should be incorporated into all such programs. These were identified as:

a) the program should be institution-wide;
b) the program should be accepted and advocated by the administration;
c) someone or some department should be given the responsibility for initiating, implementing and monitoring the activities;
d) monitoring of activities should be done using a quality assurance approach and assessment of the program should be mandatory;
e) teaching mouth-care procedures should be an integral part of all orientation and in-service programs; and
f) when developing policies with respect to mouth-care, the policy should include a description of the skills and duties or job description of those health-care workers involved, an orientation session and continuing in-service education and provision for mandatory assessment.

3. *Legislation*

It was pointed out that the functionally dependent and disabled elderly may be subject to "abuse" through the denial of needed dental services. This denial may be deliberate but it is more likely to come about through ignorance on the part of care-givers and family members. This point, therefore, should be addressed in the education section outlined above.

A further issue relates to the restricted licensing of dental hygienists to operate independently in an institutional setting. At the present time, legislation forbids dental hygienists to work unsupervised and this prevents a great deal of the much-needed preventive dental treatment from being provided to the functionally dependent and disabled elderly.

4. *Funding*

It was felt that this special population had a great need for dental services which are now largely being denied them due to a lack of funding. It was advocated that a pre-paid dental program should be introduced at the provincial level which would provide for the treatment and care of functionally dependent and disabled elderly. This was particularly important because members of this group in the population are less capable of looking after themselves.

Appendix A

Modifying Standard Preventive Approaches for the Functionally Dependent and Disabled Elderly

I. Mechanical and chemical plaque control procedures for the functionally dependent and disabled elderly

a) Is there an increasing number of functionally dependent and disabled elderly in our population?

b) Is the oral health of the functionally dependent and disabled elderly different from that of the healthy, ambulatory elderly?

c) Is the utilization of dental services influenced by the medical status of the elderly?

d) Are there mechanical and chemical plaque control procedures that have been shown to be efficacious for the functionally dependent and disabled elderly?

e) What are the problems associated with plaque control for the functionally dependent and disabled?

f) Is there a role for plaque control (mouth care) methods as a means of improving quality of life?

g) Is there a preventive program of plaque control which is appropriate for the functionally dependent and disabled elderly?

II. The role of care-givers in the oral care of the functionally dependent and disabled elderly

a) Who is the most appropriate care-giver to provide oral care?

b) Do oral care-givers require special training/education?

c) What programs are available to train oral care-givers?

d) What level of supervision is required of oral care-givers? How should performance be evaluated?

e) What community services exist to provide oral care to the functionally dependent and disabled elderly?

f) Should dental treatment be modified for the functionally dependent and disabled elderly?

g) How important do care-givers perceive oral care to be and how does this affect the oral care provided?

h) What level of oral health should we expect for the functionally dependent and disabled elderly?

III. Policies and programs of oral care for the functionally dependent and disabled elderly

   a) What policies are indicated regarding the oral health care of the functionally dependent and disabled elderly?
   b) What are the priorities with respect to oral care of the functionally dependent and disabled elderly in institutions?
   c) Who is responsible for determining policies and programs of oral care in institutions?
   d) What protocol is to be followed when a functionally dependent or disabled older adult requires oral care?
   e) What is the role of the private general dental practitioner regarding the oral care for the functionally dependent and disabled elderly? Can it be profitable?

References

Blahut P., Gerber K. and Heisch L. Efficacy of two electric toothbrushes utilized by an elderly population. *J Dent Res.* 1991;70:365, abstract 801.

Blahut P., Gerber K. and Parker W. Electric toothbrush in geriatric population, Vet. Admin. Hosp. *J Dent Res.* 1991;70:365, abstract 802.

Blahut P. and Heisch LD. Clinical evaluation of electric oral hygiene device in geriatric population. *J Dent Res.* 1991;70:365, abstract 803.

Branch LG., Antczak AA. and Stason WB. Toward understanding the use of dental services by the elderly. *Spec Care Dent.* 1986;6:38-41

Brayer L., Goultschin J. and Mor C. The effect of chlorhexidine mouthrinses on dental plaque and gingivitis in mentally retarded individuals. *Clin Prev Dent.* 1985;7:26-8.

Dane JN. The Missouri Elks mobile dental program—dental care for developmentally disabled persons. *J Pub Health Dent.* 1990;50:42-47.

Davies KW., Holloway PJ. and Worthington HV. Dental treatment for mentally handicapped adults in general practice: parents' and dentists' views. *Community Dental Health.* 1988;5:381-387.

Davies KW. and Whittle JG. Dental health education: training of homecarers of mentally handicapped adults. *Community Dental Health.* 1990;7:193-197.

DePaola. PF., Soparkar PM., Tavares M. and Kent RL Jr. The clinical profiles of individuals with and without root surface caries. *Gerodontology.* 1989;8:9-15.

Evashwick C., Rowe G. and Diehr P., et al. Factors explaining the use of health care services by the elderly. *Health Serv Res.* 1984; 19:357-382.

Friedlander AH. and Birch NJ. Dental conditions in patients with bipolar disorder on long-term lithium maintenance therapy. *Spec Care Dent.* 1990;10:148-61.

Friedlander AH. and Jarvik LF. The dental management of the patient with dementia. *Oral Surg Oral Med Oral Pathol.* 1987;64:549-53.

Gordon SR. and Sullivan TM. Dental treatment planning for compromised or elderly patients. *Gerodontics.* 1986;2:217-222.

Gilbert GH., Branch LG. and Orav EJ. Predictors of older adults' longitudinal dental care use—ten year results. *Medical Care.* 1990;28:1165-1180.

Henry R., Ownby H., Ferretti G., Brown A. and Kaplan A. Compliance of nursing personnel in administering chlorhexidine to institutionalized patients. *J Dent Res.* 1989;68:237, abstract 449.

Hunt RJ., Eldredge JB. and Beck JB. Effect of residence in a fluoridated community on the incidence of coronal and root caries in an older adult population. *J Pub Health Dent.* 1989;49:138-141.

Indresano AT. and Rooney TP. Outpatient management of mentally handicapped patients undergoing dental procedures. *J Am Dent Assoc.* 1981;102:328-330.

Jensen ME. and Kohout F. The effect of a fluoridated dentifrice on root and coronal caries in an older adult population. *J Am Dent Assoc.* 1988;117:829-832.

Jolly DE., Paulson RB., Paulson GW. and Pike JA. Parkinson's disease: a review and recommendations for dental management. *Spec Care Dent.* 1989;9:74-78.

Kalaga A., Addy M. and Hunter B. The use of 0.2% chlorhexidine spray as an adjunct to oral hygiene and gingival health in physically and mentally handicapped adults. *J Periodontol.* 1989;60:381-385.

Kenney EB., Saxe SR., Lenox JA., Cooper TM., Caudill JS. and Collins AR. The relationship of manual dexterity and knowledge to performance of oral hygiene. *J Periodontal Res.* 1976;11:67-73.

Kitamura M., Kiyak HA. and Mulligan K. Predictors of root caries in the elderly. *Community Dent Oral Epidemiol.* 1986;14:34-8.

Kiyak HA. An explanatory model of older persons' use of dental services—implications for health policy. *Medical Care.* 1987;25:936-952.

Locker D., Slade GD. and Leake JL. Prevalence of and factors associated with root decay in older adults in Canada. *J Dent Res.* 1989;68:768-772.

Nicolaci AB. and Tesini DA. Improvement in the oral hygiene of institutionalized mentally retarded individuals through training of direct care staff: a longitudinal study. *Spec Care Dent.* 1982;2:217-221.

Niessen LC. and Jones JA. Professional dental care for patients with dementia. *Gerodontology.* 1987;6:67-71.

Niessen LC. and Jones JA. Oral health and the patient with dementia. *Spec Care Dent.* 1986;6:6-12.

Niessen. LC. and Jones JA. Alzheimer's disease: a guide for dental professionals. *Spec Care Dent.* 1986;6:6-12.

Niessen LC., Jones JA., Zocchi M. and Gurian B. Dental care for the patient with Alzheimer's disease. *J Am Dent Assoc.* 1985;110:207

Persson R., Truelove E., Robinovitch M. and LeResche L. Therapeutic effects of daily chlorhexidine rinsing on oral health of a geriatric population. *Oral Surg Oral Med Oral Pathol.* 1991, in press.

Pieper K., Dirks B. and Kessler P. Caries, oral hygiene and periodontal disease in handicapped adults. *Community Dent Oral Epidemiol.* 1986;14:28-30.

Sanger RG. and Casamassimo PS. The physically and mentally disabled patient. *Dent Clin North Am.* 1983;27:363-385.

Shaw L., Shaw MJ. and Foster TD. Correlation of manual dexterity and comprehension with oral hygiene and periodontal status in mentally handicapped adults. *Community Dent Oral Epidemiol.* 1989;17:187-9.

Ship JA. Oral condition of essentially healthy patients with Alzheimer's disease. *J Dent Res.* 1989;68:306, abstract 996.

Ship JA., DeCarli C., Friedland RP. and Baum BJ. Diminished submandibular saliva flow in dementia of the Alzheimer type. *J Gerontol.* 1990;45:M61-M66.

Ship JA. and Baum BJ. Is reduced salivary flow normal in old people? *Lancet.* 1990;336:1507.

Sigal MJ., Levine N. and Barsky RL. A survey of a program for the dental care of disabled adults. *J Canada Dent Assoc.* 1988;54:1036.

Stamm JW., Banting DW. and Imrey PB. Adults root caries survey of two similar communities with contrasting natural water fluoride levels. *J Am Dent Assoc.* 1990;120:143-149.

Thornton JB., Al-Zahid S., Campbell VA., Marchetti A. and Bradley El Jr. Oral hygiene levels and periodontal disease prevalence among residents with mental retardation at various residential settings. *Spec Care Dent.* 1989;9:186-190.

Wadsworth CL., Farrington FH., Schroeder R. and Neel NL. The successes and failures of two approaches to dental care in institutions for patients who are mentally handicapped. *Spec Care Dent.* 1986;6:175-176.

Whittle JG., Grant AA. and Worthington HV. The dental health of the elderly mentally ill: a preliminary report. *Br Dent J.* 1987;162:381-383.

Yanover L., Banting DW., Grainger R. and Sandhu H. Effect of a 0.2% chlorhexidine rinse on the oral health of an institutionalized elderly population. *J Can Dent Assoc.* 1988; 595- 598.

Chapter 15
Pharmacology and Therapeutics:
The Older Periodontal Patient

Daniel A. Haas, Helen A. Grad, David L. Sumney and Michael J. Sigal

Introduction

The focus of this workshop was pharmacotherapeutics for the older patient. Proper administration of drugs to the elderly requires that we be aware of specific points which influence our approach to pharmacotherapy. This awareness involves knowing the answers to three general questions. These are:

I.   What are the underlying factors which modify pharmacotherapy for the older patient?
II. What are the specific concerns for the dental practitioner?
III. Using this information, what are our guidelines for pharmacotherapy for the elderly?

The following is a combined summary of the authors' presentations.

I. Four Factors which Modify Pharmacotherapy

Factor 1: Normal physiologic change
As we age, there are normal changes expected in our physiologic status which can lead to alterations in the way drugs act, even in the healthy older adult. These normal physiologic changes will affect both the time course of drug concentration in the body as well as the effect the drug has when it gets to its site of action. This may be restated as saying that we expect changes in both pharmacokinetics and pharmacodynamics. Therefore we must consider how these normal alterations influence the way we prescribe and administer drugs for our older patients.

Pharmacokinetics is defined as the disposition of drugs in the body. It consists of absorption, distribution, biotransformation (metabolism) and elimination.

Absorption: The impact of changes here are relatively few. There are several alterations in gastrointestinal function such as increased gastric pH, decreased gastric emptying and impaired intestinal motility. However, absorption is not an important factor unless there is specific underlying gastrointestinal disease, there has been surgical removal of part of the gastrointestinal tract, or the patient is on medication affecting gastric motility. Each of these results in aberrant absorption.

Distribution: This aspect does change in the older patient. The body components alter such that there is a decrease in lean body mass with a relative increase in adipose tissue. In males, adipose tissue increases from 18% as a young adult to 36% in later years. In females, adipose tissue increases from 33% to 48%.[1] The consequence of this change is an increase in the distribution of lipid soluble drugs such as the anxiolytic diazepam (Valium™). Therefore lipid soluble drugs will remain present in the body for longer durations, potentially resulting in a prolonged effect. As an example, the half-life for diazepam, in numbers of hours, is often stated to equal the number of years of age of that patient. This relative increase in adipose tissue also means a relative decrease in lean body mass and total body water. This results in an increase in the concentrations of drugs that are water soluble and do not distribute significantly into fatty tissues. Therefore one may find an increased potency of the drug. Drugs that are highly protein bound will have a higher free drug level in situations where albumin levels have decreased. The healthy older adult should not have alterations in plasma protein levels, but changes may occur secondary to chronic illness.

Biotransformation: The biotransformation, or metabolism, of drugs does differ in the elderly. This is a result of changes in the major organ where this takes place, the liver. Hepatic blood flow is decreased even in the healthy older adult. The ability of the Phase I enzymes to act may deteriorate with age, whereas the activity of Phase II enzymes, which conjugate compounds and thereby detoxify agents, usually is not affected. If disease is superimposed on this, a further impairment is expected. The result is a potential increase in the duration and potency of specific drugs for which biotransformation is impaired.

Elimination: Analogous to the above, differences here are a result of changes in the major organ where this takes place, the kidney. Renal clearance is decreased. Even for the healthy patient, it is expected that renal function will decrease 10% for each decade after the age of 40.[2] Other changes that occur include an age-related decrease in tubular function with respect to reabsorption, secretion and concentrating ability. The kidney is also less capable of handling acid-base imbalances.[3] Therefore the overall result of these pharmacokinetic changes is a tendency for increased duration of action and increased potency of many pharmacologic agents.

If pharmacokinetics may be defined as what the body does to drugs, *pharmacodynamics* may be defined as what the drug does to the body. Many drugs have effects that are somewhat dependent on the patients' age. In general there should be concern for agents that affect the central nervous system (CNS), such as the benzodiazepines and opioid analgesics, as their actions are often magnified in the elderly. Here one may find many psychotomimetic effects, including confusion, depression, sedation, anxiety or respiratory depression. Drugs having anticholinergic effects, as are expected with true anticholinergics such as propantheline (Probanthine™) and atropine, or antiparkinson drugs such as benztropine (Cogentin™) or trihexyphenidyl (Artane™), are of significance because of the elderly's susceptibility to these effects. Central anticholinergic effects may manifest as confusion, disorientation, poor memory and delirium.[4] Importantly, this is also a common side-effect with psychoactive drugs, which include the benzodiazepines such as diazepam (Valium™), the neuroleptics such as haloperidol (Haldol™), or tricyclic antidepressants such as amitriptyline (Elavil™). These anticholinergic effects include xerostomia, confusion or urinary retention. This latter action is a problem for males with the common finding of benign prostatic hypertrophy. Patients reporting this in their medical history should be assessed for problems with urinary retention if these anticholinergic drugs must be administered.

Factor 2: Concomitant disease
The elderly patient is much more likely to have either one or multiple systemic diseases which can further affect our pharmacotherapy. This is supported by Brasher and Rees,[5] who reported the increased incidence of systemic disease in older patients. They stated that people at age 60 or above had shown an increased prevalence of systemic problems. Reassessment of our approach to pharmacotherapy is necessary due to either the disease itself or the medications the patient is taking for its treatment. This may have a bidirectional influence in that the action of the drugs we prescribe may affect their disease, or conversely, this drug action may be affected by their disease.

Factor 3: Polypharmacy
The patient may be seeing several different medical specialists, who may not be cognizant of all of the other drugs the patient is being prescribed. The National Institute on Aging has determined that the average elderly individual takes from 4 to 5 medications at one time, and up to 20 prescriptions annually.[6] Individuals over the age of 60 represent 17% of our total population and account for 39% of all prescription drugs that are dispensed.[7] Their medications may be prescription or nonprescription. Studies indicate that the senior population of patients takes a much higher number of over-the-counter medications as compared with the general adult population.[8] One survey has noted that almost 70% of the elderly people asked used over-the-counter remedies regularly compared with 10% of the general population.[9] Multiple drugs predispose to multiple side effects that can impact on their general and oral health.

Factor 4: Drug Interactions
Polypharmacy also leads to a predisposition for interactions with the drugs we prescribe and administer. Potential for interactions increases dramatically as the number of drugs being taken increases. Adverse drug reactions are significantly more prevalent in the elderly.[10,11] It is imperative that the practitioner continually review the patient's medical history and medication list. In a study by Scully and Boyle,[12] it was reported that the direct oral interview is the most reliable approach for obtaining information. Many clinicians find the self-administered questionnaire followed by an oral review very effective for obtaining information about the medical history and medications that the patient takes.

II. Specific Concerns for the Dental Practitioner

The four factors discussed above lead to the primary concerns that we, as practitioners of dentistry, must address. These may be divided into three main areas:

1) We must know how these previous factors influence our decisions when prescribing drugs.
2) We must be aware of the side effects of systemic drugs on intraoral tissues.
3) We must be aware that some systemic agents can hamper the ability of the patient to maintain his/her own oral health.

1. Drugs We Prescribe: Analgesics and Anti-infectives.

When one looks at the potential for adverse reactions and/or interactions with drugs that a dentist would routinely prescribe, these previously mentioned factors must be considered. The presence of age-related physiologic changes, additional hepatic or renal impairment, chronic disease and medications being taken, are all important considerations. The most commonly prescribed drugs in dentistry are analgesics and anti-infectives. Therefore this section will consider the following: opioid (narcotic) analgesics, nonsteroidal anti-inflammatory drugs (NSAIDs), acetaminophen and anti-infectives.

Opioid Analgesics:
The extent and duration of analgesia produced by opioid analgesics is enhanced in the elderly patient.[13] Opioid analgesics include the following drugs in order

of potency: morphine, oxycodone (Percodan™, Percocet™), meperidine (Demerol™), pentazocine (Talwin™) and codeine. A 70-year-old patient can respond effectively to half the recommended adult dose of these opioid analgesics. The CNS is more responsive to opioids, and they are eliminated more slowly due to decreased hepatic blood flow, hepatic metabolism and renal excretion.[2] The investigation into altered renal metabolism in older patients is still in its infancy, but decreased glucuronidation of morphine by the kidney has been reported.[14] In the patient with significant hepatic or renal dysfunction, meperidine should be not be given. One of the metabolites of meperidine, normeperidine, is toxic and if it is allowed to build up can cause convulsions.[15] Substance abuse is less common in the elderly but it does exist. For example, between 2 to 10% of individuals over 60 suffer from alcoholism.[16] If the patient has a recent history of chemical dependency an opioid analgesic should be avoided. The geriatric patient may be more at risk due to the increased potency of the opioid. If an opioid analgesic is the only effective alternative it may be prescribed, but the medication should be given to the patient by a responsible third party.

Along with the enhanced analgesic efficacy of the opioids in the elderly is the increase in susceptibility to side effects, such as constipation, hypotension, dizziness, agitation, urinary retention and opioid-induced respiratory depression.[13] The constipation can be aggravated by concomitant use of the anti-ulcer medication sucralfate (Sulcrate™).[17] Postural hypotension is common in the elderly, who have additional risk factors such as diabetes, congestive heart disease or are taking anti-hypertensive medication.[18] Therefore an opioid analgesic can add to the known risk of a fall due to postural hypotension.[19] Concomitant CNS depressant medication such as the benzodiazepines, especially the long-acting sleep medication such as flurazepam (Dalmane™) or the long-acting sedatives diazepam (Valium™) or chlordiazepoxide (Librium™), can increase the risks of disorientation, sedation, falling and CNS depression in the elderly patient.[20,21] This also applies to the tricyclic anti-depressants such as amitriptyline (Elavil™), which can be used for chronic pain due to arthritis or diabetic neuropathy. Also note that gastrointestinal motility-enhancing drugs or prokinetic agents, such as metoclopramide (Maxeran™), can cause drowsiness and disorientation. The new prokinetic drug cisapride (Prepulsid™) has only a 1% incidence of such side effects.[22] The additive CNS depressant effects of alcohol and opioids will also be increased in an elderly patient due to the decrease in lean body mass.[23] Alcohol is still found in cough syrups, multiple vitamin syrups and tonics. *The Compendium of Pharmaceuticals and Specialities* has a listing of alcohol-free (less than 1%) medications.[24] The anti-ulcer medication cimetidine (Tagamet™) can increase the CNS depressant effects of opioid analgesics due to decreased metabolism, which is particularly significant in patients with renal or hepatic dysfunction.[25] Beta-adrenergic blocking agents such as propranolol (Inderal™) can also increase the toxicity of opioid analgesics and therefore have an additional effect in the elderly. Conversely, the anti-epileptic agent phenytoin (Dilantin™) decreases the effect of meperidine by increasing its metabolism.

NSAIDs:
When one looks at physiological age-related changes in the elderly it should be noted that for certain NSAIDs, namely diflunisal (Dolobid™) and naproxen (Naprosyn™), the amount of circulating free or active drug is increased by greater than 50%.[26] In addition, elderly patients are more likely to have age-related renal function impairment, which can increase the risk of NSAID-induced hepatic or renal toxicity. Therefore it is recommended by the WHO that geriatric patients, especially those over 70, be started on half the usual recommended adult NSAID dose for management of chronic pain.[13]

The use of an NSAID for analgesia in a patient with active gastrointestinal inflammatory disease is clearly contraindicated. However the question arises about the use of an NSAID analgesic in the patient with a prior history of peptic ulcer disease which was treated successfully with an anti-ulcer agent. It should be noted that there has been an increase in hospital admissions for perforated gastric and duodenal ulcers in women over 65 and men over 70 years of age. Among the factors contributing to ulcer-related complications and mortality are lack of symptoms before any serious complication.[17] Therefore the elderly patient with a prior ulcer may have developed another one but not necessarily complain of any symptoms. It is suggested that patients with a prior history of gastrointestinal inflammatory disease or with concomitant diseases which increase mortality from bleeding ulcers should be prescribed the synthetic prostaglandin E_1 analogue misoprostol (Cytotec™). It is the first drug specifically indicated for the prevention of NSAID-induced ulcers. It has been used in 500 ulcer patients over the age of 65 and found to be both safe and effective. The recommended dose is either 200 μg 4 times daily or 400 μg twice daily, taken with meals.[17]

As stated earlier, renal function decreases with age. The glomerular filtration rate (GFR) declines about 1 mL/min per year from the age of 35 to 80, renal plasma flow declines about 10% per decade and renal tubular secretory capacity declines. The decline in renal function is the single most important factor which predisposes the elderly to adverse drug reactions.[27] Doses of drugs may have to be altered if the creatinine clearance is less than 50 mL/min, or less than 0.83 mL/s in the Systeme International (SI) units.[28] However it has recently been noted that up to one-third of the elderly may have preserved near-normal GFR. In this group the assumption of decreased renal function may lead to underdosing. Therefore in robust elderly patients free of renal or cardiovascular disease, direct measurement of creatinine clearance by 24-hour urine sampling rather than usage of the standard Cockcroft and Gault formula is more accurate.[27]

In addition NSAIDs inhibit intrarenal prostaglandin production. This can decrease renal blood flow, GFR and urine volume. Indeed, a two-week course of naproxen (500 mg twice daily) in an elderly patient population resulted in a reduction of renal plasma flow by about 10%.[25] Therefore if an elderly patient requires chronic NSAID medication, the therapy should be coordinated with the physician. In elderly patients who already are dehydrated to some extent due to pre-existing cardiovascular disease, diabetes, chronic renal disease and/or diuretic therapy, the risk/benefit of long-term NSAID therapy should be critically assessed.

Short-term NSAID analgesic medication, defined as less than five days, even in a patient with pre-existing cardiovascular disease or on a diuretic medication, is perfectly acceptable.[28] In the patient with chronic renal disease, ibuprofen, which is excreted primarily via the hepatic route, would be the NSAID analgesic of choice.[29] Concurrent use of acetaminophen with diflunisal should be avoided as it may increase the acetaminophen plasma concentration by 50%, leading to acetaminophen toxicity.[30] The elderly patient will be more susceptible due to decreased hepatic function. Concurrent use of diflunisal and indomethacin has resulted in fatal gastrointestinal haemorrhage.[30] In general, the concurrent use of two NSAIDs should be avoided in the elderly patient since it greatly increases the risk of adverse effects without any significant therapeutic benefit. Levels of lithium and methotrexate, which are both drugs with a narrow therapeutic index, are increased when an NSAID is added to the patient's regimen.[30] The increase is due to a decrease in renal excretion of each drug with the addition of the NSAID. Therefore the elderly patient will be more at risk of toxicity.

Acetaminophen:
Acetaminophen analgesic doses do not have to be altered in the otherwise healthy elderly patient. However if there is suspicion the patient suffers from chronic alcoholism, therapeutic doses can cause severe hepatotoxicity. Therefore one can start with half the normal dose. Concurrent use of acetaminophen in a patient on oral anticoagulants can cause an increased anticoagulant effect. The elderly patient is more sensitive to the anticoagulant effect of warfarin, therefore one should consider using half the dose of acetaminophen and adding codeine to increase the analgesic effect.[31]

Anti-infectives:
There are no specific changes in the therapeutic use and dose of anti-infectives in otherwise healthy geriatric patients. Phenytoin levels and carbamazepine

levels can be increased in the elderly and both drugs will increase the metabolism of doxycycline—thereby rendering it ineffective. Therefore in this case one should use metronidazole and/or amoxicillin instead.[32] Erythromycin cannot be used since it decreases the hepatic metabolism of carbamazepine and this can result in toxicity in the older patient.[32] Erythromycin and ciprofloxacin also increase cyclosporin toxicity. Therefore one should weigh the risk versus benefit, and use clindamycin in this situation, if possible.[33] Tetracyclines and erythromycins can increase the levels of digoxin by decreasing its clearance. This can lead to toxicity in the elderly patient with compromised renal function (creatinine clearance less than 50 mL/min). As an alternative here one can use metronidazole or clindamycin.

Metronidazole and tetracyclines will increase levels of lithium—thereby leading to toxicity. Therefore one should avoid this combination in the geriatric renal patient. Metronidazole and ciprofloxacin will increase the anti-coagulant effect of warfarin by decreasing its hepatic metabolism.[32,33] The elderly patient is more sensitive to the anticoagulant effect of warfarin; therefore one should consider clindamycin instead. Ketoconazole will also interfere with the metabolism of warfarin; therefore one should try using a topical anti-fungal medication.[32] Ciprofloxacin interferes with the hepatic metabolism of theophylline. There have been 8 recent reports of theophylline toxicity 2 to 3 days after starting ciprofloxacin in patients between 60 to 67 years of age on therapeutic doses of theophylline.[33] Therefore one should avoid this combination.

Doxycycline can be used in elderly patients with decreased renal function but tetracycline cannot, since its use will increase blood urea nitrogen (BUN), which the kidney may be unable to handle. The dose interval should be increased for acyclovir, amoxicillin, ampicillin, cephalexin and ciprofloxacin in elderly patients with renal disease.[29]

In summary, when prescribing short-term analgesic medication, acetaminophen is still the drug of first choice. One can also consider an NSAID such as ibuprofen or flurbiprofen, with misoprostol, if necessary. If opioids need to be prescribed for the geriatric patient it is recommended to prescribe half the dose but give the patient the option of increasing the amount to a normal therapeutic dose, if necessary. For example, one could prescribe acetaminophen compound with 15 mg codeine and direct the patient to take 1 or 2 tablets every 4 to 6 hours if needed for pain. Warn the patient about possible side effects. Follow up the next day to see whether the medication is adequate and there are no significant side effects. Anti-infective therapy need not be changed in the healthy older patient.

2. Side Effects of Systemic Drugs
on Intraoral Tissues and their Management

Certain physiological and pathological tissue changes are common in dental patients who routinely take medications.[34] These changes include bruxism, gingival and periodontal disease, rampant caries, chronic caries of the root surfaces, and excessive occlusal wear patterns. Candidiasis in the oral cavity, especially under dentures, is also found frequently, as is xerostomia, glossitis, delayed wound healing, denture sores, and periodontal abscesses.[35] It is well established that there are certain changes that occur in the periodontium as individuals undergo the aging process. These changes can be visualized as gingival recession and cervical erosion at the cemento-enamel junction.[36] Experimental gingivitis has been observed to be considerably more rapid and severe in elderly people.[37] It is generally agreed that the elderly patient with moderate alveolar bone loss is more adapted to a slower progression of disease than a younger patient with the same amount of bone loss patterns at an early age.

As stated earlier, the elderly patient is more likely to be medically compromised. Due to certain pharmacological agents these patients take on a daily basis, it is extremely important to realize that there are two major possible side effects from treatment of these conditions or the use of these therapies. One of these important conditions is xerostomia. Clinical examinations of patients experiencing xerostomia show accumulations of materia alba at the cervical aspects of the teeth in the marginal gingival areas. Heavy calculus deposits and stains are usually present on the mandibular anterior teeth. Many of these patients have recurrent caries around margins of restorations and numerous areas with incipient to moderate root surface carious lesions forming. These patients usually complain of having a pasty feeling in their mouth and this condition is quite common in people over the age of fifty. Xerostomia has a definitive diagnosis that requires measurement of the salivary flow rate to be less than 0.25 mm per minute in a clinical environment. Heavy smoking, of course, precipitates a sensation like xerostomia in a number of patients already compromised by the use of required medications.

Xerostomia is a difficult condition to bring under management and many times requires consultation with physicians in order to reduce or moderate the patient's medications. The mechanical stimulation of chewing gum or foods such as carrots sometimes provides temporary relief to these patients. Alcohol-containing mouthwashes tend to increase the symptoms related to xerostomia and should be kept to a minimum. It has been proposed that pilocarpine may be of use for xerostomia associated with salivary gland dysfunction.[38] However, pilocarpine is a cholinergic agonist and may affect heart rate and blood pressure, and therefore is contraindicated in some patients. A variety of fluoride gels may be applied to the surfaces that may develop root surface caries and these are sometimes useful for preventive reasons. Patients with xerostomia should be followed quite closely and be on a routine periodontal maintenance schedule of plaque control measures and frequent dental visits. Frequent visits with these patients develop patient motivation. This also shows a positive psychological effect in that someone is listening to them and caring about this condition that causes them much discomfort and anxiety.

Oral mucositis associated with radiation therapy sometimes hinders the patient's recovery period for cancer therapy. Alleviation of severe stomatitis can provide patient comfort and facilitate a more positive attitude for recovery from cancer. In 1989, there were more than 42,000 malignant tumours of the mouth and larynx.[39] The use of appropriate mouthwashes consisting of hydrocortisone, nystatin, tetracycline, and diphenhydramine is an accepted method of controlling the discomfort of radiation-related mucositis.[40] With radiation therapy, the xerostomic condition usually diminishes in six to twelve weeks after completion of radiation therapy. Commonly, chemotherapeutic patients present with candidiasis. It is extremely useful that patients rinse with an antiseptic mouthwash and also possibly use a systemic antifungal agent. It is important to understand that in xerostomia there is a decrease in the lubricating and cleansing properties of saliva. Systemically administered ketoconazole is an effective antifungal agent which is usually well tolerated by people undergoing radiation therapy.

Older patients with xerostomia or taking xerostomic medication are at high risk for recurrent caries and root caries. In these patients, the practice of excellent oral hygiene procedures on a daily basis and the use of topical fluoride preparations is extremely beneficial. One of the most important aspects of treatment of root surface caries is to maintain a healthy intact periodontium, preventing further gingival recession, which may contribute to the development of root surface caries. Patients who must have chemotherapy and radiation therapy for the treatment of neoplasms should be seen immediately by the periodontal care team consisting of the periodontist and the hygienist. Thorough dental prophylaxis should be initiated at the beginning of treatment and accomplished at least once every four to six weeks throughout the therapy. The use of anti-plaque agents that inhibit plaque development are extremely useful in the control of cervical plaque that leads to root surface caries. The use of chlorhexidine gluconate has been established by a number of studies as an effective anti-plaque and anti-gingivitis agent. Studies have clearly shown the advantages of short-term use of chlorhexidine gluconate.[41] It is important to realize that chlorhexidine gluconate was developed for control of supragingival plaque and gingivitis prevention and not for the treatment of advanced gingivitis or periodontitis. As well, it is extremely important to realize that patients who are instructed to use chlorhexidine gluconate must also practice good oral hygiene and be a part of a total maintenance program for the control of plaque formation. The reduction of inflammation that accompanies the use of 0.12% of chlorhexidine gluconate is usually only seen in pockets less than 3 mm. In order to maximize the effects of these rinses, it is extremely important to have multiple dental prophylaxis appointments and also treat localized areas by root planing and scaling.

One of the major problems of using chlorhexidine gluconate in a periodontal maintenance program is that the patient must cooperate in its structured use. Many patients complain that the recommended usage of chlorhexidine gluconate is very expensive and produces problems of stain and increased supragingival calculus formation in the mandibular anterior areas of the teeth. However, with proper education of the patient in the many advantages of using chlorhexidine gluconate, this mouthwash is extremely beneficial in the management of plaque formation in the cervical areas of the natural dentition and the prevention of formation of root surface caries. To summarize, extensive emphasis must be placed upon the medical profile of periodontal patients and individual plaque control and maintenance programs be developed to maximize patient safety and comfort.

3. The Effect of Systemic Drugs on the Ability to Maintain Oral Health

As stated in the introduction, the elderly are managed with a diverse variety of pharmacological agents to both maintain and improve their health and well-being. Many of the medications are for the management of systemic medical conditions. However, a significant proportion are for symptomatic psychotropic therapy. The psychotropic drug group is the fifth most common family of systemic medications prescribed to the elderly. The psychotropic family of medications used in the elderly include antidepressants, anxiolytics, neuroleptics and hypnotics.[45] Elderly individuals with varying degrees of senile dementia or Alzheimer's disease would be treated symptomatically with various psychotropic agents.[42-44] In addition, many elderly with sleep disorders, depression, or anxiety attacks would also be managed with these medications.

The anxiolytics and hypnotics such as lorazepam (Ativan™), alprazolam (Xanax™), diazepam (Valium™), triazolam (Halcion™) and oxazepam (Serax™) are commonly used to control sleep disturbances associated with aging and to decrease the level of anxiety which is connected to the early stages of memory loss found in dementia, senility and Alzheimer's (42,45). However, due to a variety of pharmacokinetic and dynamic factors the medications often produce a more pronounced effect in the elderly. The individual may appear confused, ataxic, amnesic, or sedated with a decreased level of energy. The sedated individual will not be able to perform his/her own daily preventive dental care, which will thus lead to a more progressive periodontal disease status. If the individual is confused due to a drug-induced cognitive impairment he/she will not be able to perform oral hygiene adequately. The amnesic effect can also alter cognition and thus have a negative impact on oral care. Finally, the ataxia, or inability to coordinate voluntary muscle activity, will decrease their degree of self-care. Instead of ataxia developing, an oral dyskinesia can develop, which is an involuntary movement of the oral facial musculature. This can develop within days of commencing anxiolytic drug therapy. This is characterized by tongue thrusting, lip smacking, and side to side mouth movements.[45] Once the problem is noted and the medication is withdrawn it may take months before the condition resolves. As a result, oral self-care will be hindered by these uncontrolled movements and oral care provided by the dental team will be complicated by the constant motion. The final outcome will be a period of decreased oral hygiene and an exacerbation in periodontal problems. The dental team must be aware of this possible sequela of anxiolytic therapy in order to recognize it at its onset and develop modified oral hygiene measures to maintain optimum oral health during the course of anxiolytic/hypnotic therapy.[46]

If the individual is sedated, it may be easier for the primary daily attendants or dental team to perform oral hygiene procedures and sanative periodontal therapy. With this concept in mind clinicians may arrange for sedation with one of the anxiolytic/hypnotic agents for future dental appointments in order to manage their behaviour. The clinician should be aware that the elderly are very prone to developing idiosyncratic reactions to these medications. These responses include: agitation, rage, excitement and unusual behavioural patterns.[47] These idiosyncratic reactions will make the delivery of preventive dental care in a traditional clinic setting very difficult, if not impossible. In this regard, patients who do require pharmacological behaviourial management may require a general anaesthetic in order to complete any definitive dental care instead of sedation in an ambulatory clinic.

Neuroleptics such as thioridazine (Mellaril™) and haloperidol (Haldol™) are used in the treatment of hallucinations, severe agitation, delirium, and paranoid symptoms found in the elderly with dementia or Alzheimer's.[42] In addition, the neuroleptics are also commonly used for the control of dizziness, nausea, and night sedation in the elderly population.[48] It has been reported that slightly less than 2% of all the community-based elderly were taking an antipsychotic neuroleptic agent.[49] Within the Veteran's Administration Nursing Home Care Units, anywhere from 28 to 71% of the elderly patients were on antipsychotic drug therapy.[50] The utilization of these agents in the elderly population within chronic care centres is increasing. The most likely reason to explain this occurrence is that agitated, aggressive behaviour is not socially acceptable for residential living within a collective living centre.

Neuroleptics are classified as antipsychotic drugs which were originally used in the management of schizophrenia. Neuroleptic drugs antagonize the dopamine, muscarinic, histaminic and alpha-adrenergic neurotransmitter receptors to varying degrees. It is this receptor antagonism that is also responsible for their adverse effects.[51]

Neuroleptic usage by the elderly is known to produce extrapyramidal adverse effects. There are four categories of extrapyramidal symptoms, which are: dystonic reactions, pseudoparkinsonism, akathisia, and tardive dyskinesia. Approximately 50% of patients who receive haloperidol will experience extrapyramidal side effects. Dystonic reactions are characterized by an acute spasm of a muscle group, the onset of which is usually in the early stages of neuroleptic therapy. This is often seen with haloperidol. This adverse effect is reversible and will not have a significant impact on oral health. Pseudoparkinsonism, which is frequently seen in the elderly, resembles Parkinson's with a characteristic loss of facial expression and arm movements. The usual onset is after several weeks to months of neuroleptic therapy. The effect on the arms will decrease the ability of the individual to adequately perform daily oral hygiene. Therefore, these individuals will most likely have an increase in their supragingival plaque with a concomitant increase in gingival inflammation. The disorder can be treated pharmacologically, and the patient's motor control will eventually return to a more normal state. Akathisia is characterized by the patient's inability to sit still. They will demonstrate continuous agitation and restless, purposeless movements. The onset is usually after weeks of neuroleptic therapy. These movements will limit the individual's ability to perform daily oral hygiene and make it more difficult for the dental team to provide them with any form of dental care.[49,52] This will result in an increase in the prevalence and severity of periodontal disease for these individuals.

Tardive dyskinesia is the fourth extrapyramidal symptom which appears late into the course of neuroleptic drug therapy or after its withdrawal. The condition is not reversible. The prevalence of tardive dyskinesia is greater in the elderly population than in the young.[53] It has been observed that 42% of those elderly who are on neuroleptic therapy will develop dyskinesia.[54] The condition can be caused by the use of the butyrophenones such as haloperidol or the phenothiazines chlorpromazine (Largactil™), thioridazine (Mellaril™), trifluoperazine (Stelazine™) and usually develops once the dosage is decreased or the medication is withdrawn. It is believed that the disorder is the result of the development of supersensitive dopamine receptors which was caused by the chronic blockade of the receptors by the neuroleptic agents. The disorder is characterized by the development of the buccolinguomasticatory triad. This triad consists of rhythmical, involuntary movements of the tongue, lips and jaw. Clinically one observes tongue protrusion and retraction, puckering and lip smacking, and chewing movements. In addition, the individual may develop bruxism, trismus, condylar dislocation with associated facial pain, and dysphagia. The patient appears as if he/she is chewing gum or trying to reposition ill-fitting dentures. In the more severe cases there may be uncontrolled, rhythmical movement of the trunk, fingers, toes, arms, and legs.[48,55-57] Patients are often unaware of these movements, and if they try to suppress them, they can only do so for a short period of time.

These uncontrolled movements of the masticatory system will make it extremely difficult for the patient to maintain an adequate level of oral hygiene. Therefore, plaque will accumulate and gingival inflammation will develop. The uncontrolled movements will also limit the degree of oral care that the dental team can provide to the individual. In extreme cases, a general anaesthetic may be used to complete a thorough examination and to perform any treatment that is required, which would include periodontal therapy.

The dentist should also be aware that the uncontrolled movements of the masticatory system may result in dysphagia, which will then render the patient more prone to choking and possible aspiration. This can occur during dental treatment; so the clinician must be careful when using copious irrigation such as that employed with ultrasonic scalers, prophyjets, and high-speed drills, in order to prevent possible aspiration. High-volume suction and positioning of the patient in a more upright posture will decrease the potential for aspiration.

This section has outlined how certain psychotropic medications that are commonly prescribed for the elderly can decrease the ability of the individual to maintain their own level of oral hygiene, and make it more difficult for the dentist/attendant to provide the required oral maintenance care to them. As a result, the elderly will have an increased incidence of periodontal problems, which are usually very difficult to reverse. The dentist who is treating the elderly must be aware of medications which by altering the patient's mood or psychological state can have an adverse effect of their periodontal status.

Therefore, using all the above information, we conclude by considering the guidelines for pharmacotherapy for the older patient.

III. Guidelines to Pharmacotherapy for the Older Patient

1. Simplify.

As the older patient is predisposed to this array of problems, it is imperative that we keep our pharmacotherapy simple. In so doing, we will minimize the likelihood for adverse reactions and interactions. Everything else should follow logically from this. As a generality, one should avoid drugs with long durations, those with prominent CNS effects or relatively new drugs. The potential problem with the relatively new medications is that they are often primarily tested in young, healthy adults and adverse effects may not be seen until sufficient numbers have taken the drug to result in reports of toxicity.

2. Decrease the number of drugs.
This is part of the approach of simplification. Give only as few as are needed to accomplish the treatment.

3. Decrease the initial dose of drugs.
Due to the pharmacokinetic and pharmacodynamic changes, drugs often have exaggerated effect, especially those acting on the CNS. Therefore, initially give 50% of the usual dose.

4. Decrease the frequency of drug administration.
Because the pharmacokinetic changes often lead to an increased duration of action, recommended frequencies may be inappropriate. As an example, instead of every 4 hours, consider every 6 or 8.

5. Monitor.
We must monitor the patient to assess if our decisions on dose and frequency were appropriate. This monitoring should involve follow-up both in the short term (that day) and longer term (that week).

6. Review the medication list.
These patients may continually have their drugs changed by their physicians, especially if they are being seen by multiple specialists, as is often the case. In order to make the correct pharmacotherapeutic decisions, you must be aware of the accurate list of medications the patient is taking.

7. Look for the oral manifestations of these drugs.
These are most often seen as xerostomia, leading to root caries. If present consider treatment with fluoride gels or chlorhexidine applications.

8. *Look for psychoactive drug-induced impairment of the patients' ability to maintain oral health.*

Be aware that because of the side effects of certain systemic psychoactive drugs, the patient may not be able to maintain oral health. You may have to ensure that someone is attending to this need of the patient.

9. *Consider consulting with the physician to reduce the dose of the psychoactive drug if you perceive the side effects to be significantly debilitating.*

This should be a natural part of your responsibility as a provider of health care.

Endnotes

1.   Carty MA, Everitt DE. Basic principles of prescribing for geriatric outpatients. *Geriatrics.* 1989; 44:85-98.
2.   Beers MH, Ouslander JG. Risk factors in geriatric drug prescribing, a guide to avoiding problems. *Drugs.* 1989; 37:105-112.
3.   Paul MD. Renal disease in the elderly. *Medicine North America.* 1988; 28:5261-5236.
4.   Sternberg SK. Drug interactions in the elderly: which are significant? *Geriatric Medicine.* 1986; 2:9-11.
5.   Brasher, WJ, Rees, TD. Systemic conditions in the management of periodontal patients. *J. Periodontol.* 1970; 41:349.
6.   Lamy PP. Pharmacotherapeutics in the elderly. *Maryland Med. J.* 1989; 38:144-148.
7.   Baum C, Kennedy, DL, Knapp DE, Juergens JP, Faich GA. Prescription drug use in 1984 and changes over time. *Med. Care.* 1988; 26:105-114.
8.   Guttman, D. Patterns of legal drug use by older Americans. *Addict. Dis.* 1977; 3:337.
9.   Steinberg JR Prescription drug impairment in the elderly. *Drug Therapy.* 1990; Suppl 83-100.
10.   Montamat SC, Cusack BJ, Vestal RE. Management of drug therapy in the elderly. *New England Journal of Medicine.* 1989; 321:303-309.
11.   Gordon M. Principles in prescribing for the older patient. *Drug Protocol.* 1987; 2:15-24.
12.   Scully, C, Boyle, P. Reliability of a self-administered questionnaire for screening medical problems in dentistry. *Comm. Dent. Oral Epidemiol.* 1983; 11:105.
13.   Enck RE. Pain control in the ambulatory elderly. *Geriatrics.* 1991; 46:49-58.
14.   Dawling S, Crome P. Clinical pharmacokinetic considerations in the elderly. *Clin. Pharmacokin.* 1989; 17:236-56.
15.   Sanders HD. Polypharmacy in the elderly. *Can. Fam. Physician.* 1991; 37:120-124.
16.   Jinks MJ and Raschko RR. A profile of alcohol and prescription drugabuse in a high risk community-based elderly population. *DICP.* 1990; 971-975
17.   Freston MS and Freston JW. Peptic ulcers in the elderly: unique features and management. *Geriatrics.* 1990; 45:39-42.
18.   Rosenthal MJ and Naliboff B. Postural hypotension: its meaning and management in the elderly. *Geriatrics.* 1988; 43:31-40.
19.   Gryfe CI and Gryfe-Becker BM. The association of drugs with falls among the elderly. *Can Pharm J.* 1986; 119:201-03.

20. Conrad KA. Sedative hypnotic drug use in the elderly. *Drug Therapy.* 1990; 20:22-27

21. Smith DA. New rules for prescribing psychotropics in nursing homes. *Geriatrics.* 1990; 45:44-56.

22. Kauvax D and Brandt LJ. Treatment of common GI disorders in the elderly. *Drug Therapy.* 1991; 21:23-34.

23. Cadieux RJ. Drug Interactions in the elderly. *Postgrad. Med.* 1989; 86:179-86.

24 Krogh CME, ed. *Compendium of pharmaceuticals and specialties.* Ottawa: Canadian Pharmaceutical Assoc., 1990:B4.

25. Brawn LA and Castleden CM. Adverse drug reactions an overview of special considerations in the management of the elderly patient. *Drug Safety.* 1990; 5:421-35.

26. Wallace SM and Verbeeck RK. Plasma protein binding of drugs in the elderly. *Clin. Pharmacokin.* 1987;12:41-72.

27. Lonergan ET. Aging and the kidney: Adjusting treatment to physiologic change. *Geriatrics.* 1988; 43:27-33.

28. Gurwitz JH, Avorn J, Ross-Degnan D, Lipsitz LA. Nonsteroidal anti-inflammatory drug-associated azotemia in the very old. *JAMA.* 1990; 264:471-75.

29. Cove-Smith R. Drugs and the kidney. *Medicine International.* 1991;85:3539-3546.

30. United States Pharmacopeial Convention.*Drug information for the health care professional.* Rockville, MD: USP, 1991:11:474-82.

31. Harrington R and Ansell J. Risk-benefit assessment of anticoagulant therapy. *Drug Safety.* 1991; 6:54-69.

32. Rizack MA, Hillman CDM. Handbook of adverse drug interactions. *The Medical Letter.* New York, 1989.

33. Paton JH and Reeves DS. Clinical features and management of adverse effects of quinolone antibacterials. *Drug Safety.* 1991; 6:8-27.

34. Brightman, VJ: Dental Correlations: Alcohol and Drug Abuse. In Rose, LF and Kaup, D, eds. *Internal Medicine for Dentistry.* St. Louis, C.V. Mosby, 1983; 862.

35. Rees, TD. Dental Management of the medically compromised patient. In McDonald, RE, Hurt, WC, Gilmore, HW and Middleton, RA, eds. *Current Therapy in Dentistry.* St. Louis, C.V. Mosby, 1980; 21.

36. Tonna, EA. Factors affecting bone and cementum. *J. Periodontol.* 1976, 47:267-280.

37. Holm-Pedersen, P, Agerback, N, and Theilade, R. Experimental gingivitis in young and elderly individuals.*J. Clin. Periodontol.* 1975, 2:14-26.

38. Fox, PC, Vander Van, PF, Baum, BJ, and Mandel, ID. Pilocarpine for the treatment of xerostomia associated with salivary gland dysfunction. *Oral Surg.* 1986, 61:243-248.
39. Chen, TY, Webster, JH. Oral monilia study on patients with head and neck cancer during radiotherapy. *Cancer.* 1974, 34:246-249.
40. Rothwell, BR and Spektor, WS. Palliation of radiation-related mucositis. *Special Care in Dentistry.* 1990, 10:21-25.
41. Greenstein, G, Berman, C and Jaffin, R. Chlorhexidine—An adjunct to periodontal therapy. *J. Periodontol.* 1986, 57:370-377.
42. Fujimoto-Thompson D, Shimomura SK. Alzheimer's disease (Primary degenerative dementia of the Alzheimer type). In: Herfindel ET, Gourley DR, Hart LL, eds. *Clinical Pharmacology and Therapeutics.* Baltimore; Williams and Wilkins, 1988:652-660.
43. Seltzer B. Dementia: Its diagnosis and medical management. *Gerodontol.* 1987; 6:47-52.
44. Somerman MJ. Dental implications of pharmacological management of the Alzheimer's patient. *Gerodontol.* 1987; 6:59-65.
45. Strauss A. Oral dyskinesia associated with buspirone use in elderly woman. *J. Clin. Psychiatry.* 1988; 49:322-323.
46. Culberston VL. The clinical pharmacology and dental use of benzodiazepines in the elderly. *Gerodontics.* 1985; 1:252-260.
47. Hall R, Zisook S. Paradoxical reactions to benzodiazepines. *Br. J. Clin. Pharmacol.* 1981; 11:99-104.
48. Pall HS, William AC. Extrapyramidal disturbances caused by inappropriate prescribing. *Brit. Med. J.* 1987; 295:30-31.
49. Mellinger G, Balter M. Prevalence and patterns of use of psychotherapeutic drugs: Results from a 1979 national survey of American adults. In: Tognoni G, Ballantuono C, Lader M, eds. *Epidemiological impact of psychotropic drugs.* Amsterdam: Elsevier, 1981:117-135.
50. Custer R, Davis J, Gee S. Psychiatric drug usage in VA nursing home care units. *Psychiatr. Ann.* 1984; 14:285-292.
51. Stimmel GL. Schizophrenia. In: Herfindal ET, Gourley DR, Hart LL, eds. *Clinical pharmacology and therapeutics.* Baltimaore: Williams and Wilkins, 1988:639-651.
52. Dickey W, Morrow JI. Drug induced neurological disorders. *Prog. in Neurobiology.* 1990; 34:331-342.
53. Johnson GFS, Hunt GE, Rey JM. Incidence and severity of tardive dyskinesia increase with age. *Arch. Gen. Psychiatry.* 1982; 39:486.
54. Bourgeois M, Bouilh P, Tignol J, Yesavage JA. Spontaneous dyskinesias vs. neuroleptic-induced dyskinesias in 270 elderly subjects. *J. Nerv. Ment. Dis.* 1980; 168:177-178.

55.   Levy SM, Baker KA, Semia TP, Kohout FJ. Medications with dental significance, use by a non-institutionalized elderly population. *Geriodontics.* 1988; 4:119-125.

56.   Baker KA, Ettinger RL. Intra-oral effects of drugs in elderly persons. *Geriodontics.* 1985; 1:111-116.

57.   Osborne TE, Grace EG, Schwartz MK. Severe degenerative changes of the temporomandibular joint secondary to the effects of tardive dyskinesia: a literature review and case report. *J. Craniomand. Pract.* 1989; 7:58-62.

Chapter 16
Educational Models for Teaching Periodontal Care for Older Adults

Ronald L. Ettinger, Paul B. Robertson, Peter Birek, and Mai Pohlak.

Introduction

An Older Adult can be described as being the sum total of his or her life experience. Similarly, the oral status of an older adult is the sum total of his or her life experience with systemic diseases which have oral manifestations, with dental diseases which include caries and periodontal disease as well as iatrogenic disease.[1] Oral status is also influenced significantly by the attitudes, skills, and philosophies of the dentists he or she has encountered. In the not so recent past, the elderly as well as the dental profession had stereotyped the aging population as being primarily edentulous and thus in need only of removable prosthodontics services.[2] As recently as 1985, Braun and Marcus[3] found that dentists who participated in a treatment planning experiment increased the extraction rate and decreased the use of fixed prosthodontics for patients aged 60 years and older when compared with similar oral problems in younger patients. The need for periodontal care in such an environment was irrelevant. However, the documented changes in caries[4-6] as well as the reduction in tooth loss[7-10] has resulted in the emergence of a new older dental consumer who will not accept tooth loss as inevitable and seeks to maintain his or her dentition.[2] These patients bring with them complex oral and treatment problems, a few of which are listed below:

1. exposed furcations
2. radicular grooves
3. split roots
4. root surface restorations
5. restoration below the gingival margin.

How does one teach periodontal care to such a population when they may also be handicapped by:

1. poor eyesight
2. loss of fine motor skills
3. use of multiple medications, many with xerostomic potential
4. progressive cognitive impairment
5. ill health
6. problems with transportation and a
7. reduced ability to learn the new neuromuscular skills.

It is the purpose of this paper to address some of the issues which may help to develop strategies to deal with these problems.

The principles of caring for the periodontium are to prevent the loss of periodontal attachment. This loss is usually caused by microorganisms which have colonized the teeth. In general, bone loss in periodontal disease is irreversible, although significant advances have been made in the treatment and regeneration of lost periodontal supporting structures.[11-13] Traditionally, the successful outcome of care depended upon the cooperation of the patient and/or their significant other and the clinician in maintaining an adequate level of personal hygiene. How to achieve the goal of plaque reduction in an aging population is the basis of this discussion.

Before one can discuss the issues of treating periodontal disease there are some questions and problems associated with an aging population which need to be highlighted.

Firstly —   Periodontal disease can be:
1. insidious
2. usually asymptomatic
3. poorly understood by the public and
4. difficult for the public to recognize.

If that is the case, how does one motivate the public to seek care, to learn new neuromuscular skills and to accept the treatment regimen suggested by the dentist?

Secondly — The traditional continuous destructive disease model of periodontal disease has been replaced in most peoples' minds with the "burst model" which stresses the fact that severe periodontal disease occurs only in a few sites in a relatively small number of people.[14-17]
1. If this is so, is the traditional way of preventing periodontal disease by targeting individual behaviour modification appropriate?
2. If not, how can one identify the high risk group? and
3. How can one develop strategies to target the problems of the high risk group and have them come to seek treatment?

Thirdly —   Evidence suggests that in general the more plaque a person has the more likely they are to have more disease, although the type of microorganisms in the plaque have considerable influence on the pathogenesis of the disease.[18-20] Nevertheless, to reduce plaque in the general population must be the aim of any program.

1. If that is the case one must begin to understand why some people have high plaque scores and other low plaque scores.
2. Also it is not known what effect psycho-social events have on a person's immune response, e.g., divorce, unemployment, retirement, bereavement, etc.

Overriding all of periodontal care is the fact that even with oral health awareness that leads an individual to the use of dental services, these services will always be subject to economic restraint, and more recently the limits are being set by a third party payment providers.

Keeping some of these issues in mind educational models for teaching periodontal health for older adults must target the dental student, the dental profession, the patients themselves and also the patients' caregivers, be they significant others or health care providers.

Interdisciplinary Models

The complex medical and pharmacotherapeutic history of many older patients will require an interdisciplinary approach. The problems of this group of individuals have been associated with salivary gland dysfunction, sensory disorders, an often incomplete dentition that is heavily restored, and physical disabilities that compromise the patients' ability to maintain adequate oral hygiene. For such patients, neither their systemic dysfunction nor their oral lesions respect the traditional mucogingival boundary between the provinces of oral medicine and periodontics.

In an essay on postdoctoral periodontics training, Hurt[21] argues that clinical and didactic experience in oral medicine, a discipline that deals with the interrelationships between oral and systemic disease, is increasingly important to the delivery of periodontal care. Indeed, he notes that the two disciplines were once interrelated and that a renewed marriage of clinical oral medicine and periodontics would be healthy and appropriate. Therefore, it may be in the best interest of students as well as the profession to merge these two disciplines.

There is considerable evidence that the etiology of gingivitis and periodontitis is microbial plaque, and that the inflammatory lesion will not occur in the absence of microorganisms. However, many forms of gingivitis and periodontitis have been related to the establishment of a pathogenic microflora in a systemically compromised host. A higher prevalence of gingivitis has been associated with a variety of systemic diseases[22-25] including acute leukaemia, Addison's disease, diabetes, haemophilia, thrombocytopenia, sclerosis, Sturge-Weber syndrome, Wegener's granulomatosis, and combined immunodeficiency diseases. Acute necrotizing ulcerative gingivitis is often seen among individuals with impaired host defence mechanisms associated with stress, malnutrition, and a variety of systemic diseases, as well as patients with acquired and therapeutically induced immunosuppression.[26-28] Gingival enlargement or overgrowth is a well documented side effect of several drugs, particularly phenytoin, cyclosporin, and nifedipine.[29-31] Forms of gingivitis associated with hormonal changes are characterized by exaggerated inflammatory responses to microbial plaque, with severe redness, edema, bleeding and enlargement.[32-34] The disease is seen primarily in pregnancy but similar gingival changes have also been reported with puberty, the menstrual cycle, steroid therapy, and menopause.[35-38] The pathogenesis of hormonally influenced gingival lesions has been related to the profound effect of steroid levels on both the gingival microvasculature and the subgingival microflora.[39-41] HIV-associated gingivitis (HIV-G) has been reported in 15% to 50% of patients with acquired immunodeficiency syndrome (AIDS) associated with the human immunodeficiency virus (HIV).[42-44] The microbial profile of sites exhibiting HIV-G[45-48] is similar to forms of periodontitis, but substantially different than gingivitis and, in addition, may include high proportions of *Candida albicans*.

Most of the early-onset and rapidly progressing forms of periodontitis are associated with systemic disturbances, particularly defects in neutrophil function. Severe periodontitis has also been observed in other primary neutrophil disorders[49-52] including agranulocytosis, cyclic neutropenia, and Chédiak-Higashi, Job's and lazy leukocyte syndromes. In addition, periodontitis is reported as more frequent and severe in diabetes, Down's syndrome, Papillon-LeFèvre syndrome, inflammatory bowel diseases and Addison's disease, which exhibits secondary or associated neutrophil impairment.[24,25,53,55] Unusual forms of periodontitis are more frequent in severe combined and acquired immunodeficiency diseases.[56] Rapidly progressive periodontitis shares many of the features of generalized juvenile periodontitis including severe gingival inflammation, rapid loss of alveolar bone and, in many subjects, depressed neutrophil function.[57] HIV-associated periodontal lesions may predispose to necrotizing stomatitis, an acute, massively destructive ulcerative and necrotizing lesion of the gingiva that extends into contiguous mucosal and osseous tissues.[60]

While the accumulation of microorganisms and associated gingival inflammation appear to be a prerequisite,[61-63] mechanisms responsible for the transition or conversion of gingivitis to periodontitis remain largely unclear. However, there is substantial evidence that host systems play a major role. A number of host disturbances have been proposed that could serve to facilitate the colonization and subsequent dominance of a pathogenic microflora.[64-68] Once established, these organisms appear to incite destruction of the supporting structures by both direct toxic effects on adjacent tissues and, in greater measure, by indirect activation of host cells to produce a variety of acute inflammatory mediators, arachidonic acid metabolites, cytokines, phagocyte granule components, reactive oxygen species, and collagenolytic enzymes. Moreover, these microorganisms are capable of interfering with mechanisms that control the neutrophil-antibody-complement and lymphocyte-macrophage-cytokine axes of the host defense system. These host disturbances important to etiology and host mechanisms responsible for pathogenesis of the periodontal diseases are affected by the aging process,[69] and are equally relevant to disciplines concerned with diseases of the periodontium and relationships between oral and systemic disease.

The Medical Model

The complexity of care of frail older adults suggests that possibly the best way to educate dental students to care for these patients is to use the Medical Model. That is, patients are assigned to a specific instructor, who works with a group of students for a defined period of time. The student delivers the care to the patient under the supervision of the faculty member. When the student completes his rotation the patient remains the responsibility of the faculty instructor and, if necessary, dental treatment progresses with a new group of students. The Iowa experience[70-72] over the last ten years has suggested that these frail older adults are best treated in a clinic which is designed for their needs. This includes easy access, separate waiting room, toilets available near the clinic area, trained dental assistants and clinic clerks who are prepared to deal with family, institutions and government agencies. The students should be senior students who are confident enough of their clinical skills not to be overwhelmed by the complexities of the medical problems and pharmaco-therapies.[71] Such programs also will require a trained cadre of clinical teachers in each dental school and postgraduate training facility.

Dental Hygienists

The dental hygienist will play an increasingly important role in the maintenance of care for older adults as more and more older adults retain their dentitions. This will be particularly significant for the care of functionally dependent older adults living in long term care institutions, be they nursing homes or hospitals.

To be able to achieve this goal will require some changes in legislation in certain states or provinces as well as a significant increase in the teaching of oral medicine and pharmacology in hygiene schools. It will also require hands-on experience in long term care institutions for the dental hygiene students.

Interceptive Geriatrics

As the numbers of older dentate adults increase, the manpower required to treat their increasing needs may overwhelm scarce resources. It would seem wiser to think towards the future and campaign not towards the treatment of all potential disease but rather towards the development of a preventive philosophy which one might call "Interceptive Geriatrics." The simplest explanation might be to use the example of an individual who has just been diagnosed with Alzheimer's disease. The projected lifespan of this person is about 10 years while a progressive deterioration occurs.[73] When caring for such a patient the philosophy of care is to treat oral disease aggressively early and institute practical preventive procedures.[74-77] Such a treatment plan would include the extraction of teeth with poor prognosis and their subsequent replacement if necessary with fixed or removable prostheses. The institution of preventive procedures such as home use fluorides and frequent recalls would be helpful. These appointments should involve the patients' significant others because they will become the caregivers. For functionally independent older adults such a philosophy of "interceptive geriatrics" need not be quite so aggressive but would follow similar principals. This will require a treatment decision philosophy sensitive to the prospective medical/psychological condition of the patient as well as the constraints imposed by finances. Such rational treatment planning, which tries to predict treatment outcome, should be the basis for any educational model which addresses this issue of oral health care for older adults.

The Functionally Dependent Older Adult

The most difficult group to plan for are functionally dependent older adults living in long term care institutions, because their oral health maintenance care is often dependent on their caregivers. Most oral health problems, including periodontal disease, are not life-threatening conditions and so treatment is not deemed important enough to fit into a collaborative model of health care. It is imperative that dental professionals initiate and teach how good oral health care can affect the quality of a resident's life.

Personal oral hygiene requires the removal of plaque and if residents can do it independently they should be encouraged to do so. For those residents who can no longer take responsibility for their own oral health care another individual must take over to serve the best interest of the resident. Ideally that person should be a dentist or a dental hygienist but in reality it is usually a nurse's aide. The model shown in Figure 1 is a conceptual educational model aimed at these caretakers.

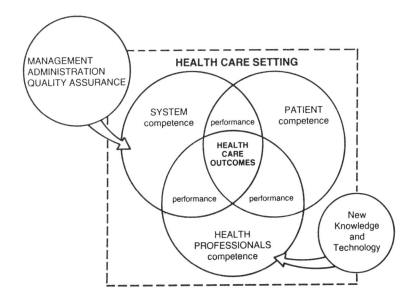

Figure 1 — Conceptual Model for Education of Health Professionals

Programs to educate caregivers can be effective only through changing behaviours of the individual health professionals. As adult learners, these individuals have clear ideas about what the issues, concerns and problems are in their professional lives. For the staff development program to be successful, those individuals who participate must feel an involvement in, commitment to and responsibility for the design, content and the process of learning.[79] Full involvement of all participants will ensure that the activity is focused on real life concerns and therefore be seen as meaningful and relevant to the participants. Thus the education program originates from the health care setting—a complex system composed of patients' health care delivery system and the function of the health care professional.

Often the caregivers themselves have poor oral health and poor knowledge of how to deliver oral health care. Therefore, providing caregivers with a sound knowledge base in periodontal care and oral hygiene measures may not immediately result in behavioral changes in their patients but may have some other spin-off effects.[78] The caregivers themselves may change their oral health behaviours, and once comfortable with the changes, they may readily and more willingly incorporate preventive oral health care regimens in their daily health care activities with the seniors. Even if changes cannot be expressed in measurable terms but only in vague perceptions, changes in health care behaviours and outcomes are the ultimate goals of any educational program.[80]

The responsibility of the dental professional is to serve as a facilitator and a resource person. While the staff caregivers will become responsible for daily oral hygiene care for the functionally dependent older adult, the dental professional remains as a consultant to the oral hygiene maintenance program, collecting and disseminating resource materials, providing and receiving feedback on progress and assessing the outcomes of care in terms of health status and well being of the patients. The driving force in this learning process is motivation, rooted in the health professional's sense of responsibility, and the rewards of this process will be seen in the transformation of the potential state of the art of dental health care into actual health care outcomes.[81,82]

In summary, the health care activities in any collective living centre will emphasize individual patient's and society's values and preferences and are oriented towards desired outcomes. Quality assurance in a given institution is the joint responsibility of administration, health care professionals, patients and support staff. The inter-relationship of structure, process and outcomes will determine the quality of life and welfare of the individuals trusted in the care of that institution.[78]

Endnotes

1.   Ettinger, R.L. Restoring the aging dentition: Repair or Replacement? *Int Dent J.* 1990; 40:275-282.

2.   Ettinger, R.L. Beck, J.D. The new elderly: what can the dental profession expect? *Spec Care Dent.* 1982; 2:62-69.

3.   Braun R.J. Marcus M. Comparing treatment decision for elderly and young dental patients. *Gerodontics.* 1989; 1:138-142.

4.   Katz RV, Hazen SP, Chilton NW, Mumma D. Prevalence and intraoral distribution of root caries in an adult population. *Caries Res.* 1982; 16:265-271.

5.   Bohannan HM. The impact of decreasing caries prevalence: Implications for dental education. *J Dent Educ.* 1982; 61:1369-1377.

6.   Graves RC Stamm JW. Oral health status in the United States: Prevalence of dental caries. *J Dent Educ.* 1985; 49:341-345.

7.   Weintraub JA Burt BA. Oral health status in the United States: Tooth loss and edentulism. *J Dent Educ.* 1985; 49:368-376.

8.   Beck JD Hunt RJ. Oral health status in the United States: Problems of special patients. *J Dent Educ.* 1985; 49:407-425.

9.   U.S. Department of Health and Human Services. Oral health of United States Adults. National findings. *N.I.H. Publication No. 87-2868*, August 1987.

10.   Hunt RJ, Hand JS, Kohout FJ, Beck JD. Incidence of tooth loss among elderly Iowans. *Am J Pub Hlth.* 1988; 78:1330-1332.

11.   Hirsch RS, Clark NG. Differential diagnosis of severe periodontal disease. *Aust Dent J.* 1989; 34:548-558.

12.   Ciancio SG. Agents for the management of plaque and gingivitis. *J Am Coll Dent.* 1989; 56:14-20.

13.   Smith PG Seymour RA. Periodontal disease and treatment in the elderly: 2. *Dent Update* 1989; 16:50-55.

14.   Lindhe J, Haffajee AD, Socransky SS. Progression of periodontal disease in adult subjects in the absence of periodontal therapy. *J Clin Periodontol.* 1983; 10:435-42.

15.   Haffajee AD, Socransky SS, Goodson JM. Clinical parameters as predictors of destructive periodontal disease. *J Clin Periodontol.* 1983; 10:257-65.

16.   Becker W, Berg L, Becker BE. Untreated periodontal disease: A longitudinal study. *J Periodontol.* 1983; 10:453:42.

17.   Socransky, SS, Haffajee, AD, Goodson JM, Lindhe J. New concepts of destructive periodontal disease. *J Clin Periodontol.* 1984; 11:21-32.

18.   Holm-Pedersen P, Folke LEA, Gawronsi TH. Composition and metabolic activity of dental plaque from healthy young and elderly individuals. *J Dent Res*. 1980; 59:771-776.
19.   Lindhe J, Nyman S. The effect of plaque control and surgical pocket elimination as the establishment and the maintenance of periodontal health. A longitudinal study of periodontal therapy in cases of advanced disease. *J Clin Periodontol*. 1975; 2:67-79.
20.   Page RC. Current understanding of the aetiology and progression of periodontal disese. *Int Dent J*. 1986; 36:153-161.
21.   Hurt WC, Clinical oral medicine. An exciting facet of postdoctoral periodontic training. *J Periodontol*. 1986; 57:426-428.
22.   Page RC. Gingivitis. J Clin Periodontol 1986; 13:345-539.
23.   Genco RJ, Zambon JJ, Christersson LA. The origin of periodontal infections. *Adv Dent Res*. 1988; 2:245-259.
24.   Genco RJ, Slots J. Host responses in periodontal disease. *J Dent Res*. 1984; 63:441-451.
25.   Rees T. Adjunctive therapy. In: Nevins M, Becker W, Kornman K. *Proceedings of the World Workshop in Clinical Periodontics*. American Academy of Periodontology. 1989:X-1.
26.   Cogen RB. Acute necrotizing ulcerative gingivitis. In: Genco RJ, Goldman HM, Cohen DW, eds. *Contemporary Periodontics*. St. Louis: C.V. Mosby, 1990:459-465.
27.   Silverman S Jr., Migliorati CA, Lozada-Nur F, Greenspan D, Conant MA. Oral findings in people with or at high risk for AIDS: A study of 375 homosexual males. *J Am Dent Assoc*. 1986; 112:187-92.
28.   Schiodt M, Pinborg JJ. AIDS and the oral cavity. Epidemiology and clinical oral manifestations of human immune virus infection. *Int J Oral Maxillofac Surg*. 1987; 16:1-14.
29.   Hassell T. *Epilepsy and the oral manifestations of phenytoin therapy*. Basel, Switzerland: S Karger; 1981.
30.   Rateitschak-Pluss EM, Hefti A, Lortscher R, Thiel G. Initial observation that cyclosporin-A induces gingival enlargement in man. *J Clin Periodontol*. 1983; 10:237-246.
32.   Löe H, Silness J. Periodontal disease in pregnancy. I Prevalence and Severity. *Acta Odontol Scand*. 1963; 21:532-551.
33.   Cohen DW, Friedman L, Shapiro J, Kyle GC. A longitudinal investigation of the periodontal changes during pregnancy. *J Periodontol*. 1969; 40:563-570.
34.   Cohen DW, Shapiro J, Friedman L, Kyle GC, Franklin S. A longitudinal investigation of the periodontal changes during pregnancy and fifteen months post-partum. Part II. *J Periodontol*. 1971; 42:653-657.

35. El-Shiry GM, El-Kafrawy AH, Nasr MF, Younis N. Efects of oral contraceptives on the gingiva. *J Periodontol.* 1971; 42:273-275.

36. Knight GM, Wade AB. The effects of hormonal contraceptives on the human periodontium. *J Periodont Res.* 1974; 9:18-22.

37. Kalkwarf KL. Effect of oral contraceptive therapy on gingival inflammation in humans. *J Periodontol.* 1978; 49:560-563.

38. Lindhe J, Bjorn AL. Influence of hormonal contraceptives on the gingiva of women. *J Periodont Res.* 1967; 2:1-6.

39. Lindhe J, Branemark PI. The effects of sex hormones on vascularization of granulation tissue. *J Periodont Res.* 1968; 3:611-619.

40. Mohamed AH, Waterhouse JP, Freiderici HHR. The microvasculature of the rabbit gingiva as affected by progesterone: An ultrastructural study. *J Periodontol.* 1974; 45:50-60.

41. Kornman KS, Loesche WJ. The subgingival microbial flora during pregnancy. *J Periodont Res.* 1980; 15:111-122.

42. Gornitsky M, Pekovic D. Involvement of human immunodeficiency virus (HIV) in gingiva of patients with AIDS. *Adv Exp Med Biol.* 1987; 216A:553-562.

43. Schulten EA, ten Kate RW, van der Waal I. Oral Manifestations of HIV infection in 75 Dutch Patients. *J Oral Pathol Med.* 1989; 18:42-46.

44. Porter SR, Luker J, Scully C, Glover S, Griffiths MJ. Oral manifestations of a group of British patients infected with HIV-1. *J Oral Pathol Med.* 1989; 18:47-48.

45. Murray PA, Winkler JR, Sadowski L, et al. Microbiology of HIV-associated gingivitis and periodontitis. In: Robertson PB, Greenspan JS, eds. *Perspectives on Oral Manifestations of AIDS.* San Diego, Calif. Littleton, Mass.: PSG Publishing Co., Inc. 1988-105.

46. Murray Pa, Grassi M, Winkler JR. The microbiology of HIV-associated periodontal lesions. *J Clin Periodontol.* 1989; 16:636-642.

47. Murray PA, Winkler JR, Peros WJ, French CK, Lippke JA. DNA probe detection of periodontal pathogens in HIV-associated periodontal lesions. *Oral Microbiol Immunol.* 1991; 6:34-40

48. Zambon JJ. Overview of the microbiology of periodontal disease. In: Robertson PB, Greenspan JS, eds. *Perspectives on Oral Manifestations of AIDS.* San Diego, Calif. Littleton, Mass. PSG Publishing Co., Inc. 1988; 296.

49. Van Dyke TE, Offenbacher S, Place D, Dowell VR, Jones J. Refractory periodontitis: Mixed infection with Bateroides gingivalis and other unusual Bacteroides species. A case report. *J Periodontol.* 1988; 59:189.

50. Van Dyke TE, Levine MJ, Genco RJ. Periodontal diseases and neutrophil abnormalities. In: Genco RJ, Mergenhagen SE, eds. *Host-Parasite Interactions in Periodontal Diseases.* Washington, D.C.: American Society for Microbiology. 1982; 235.

51. Cohen DW, Morris AL. Periodontal manifestations of cyclic neutropenia. *J Periodontol.* 1961; 32:159-168.

52. Tempel TR, Kimball HR, Kakehashi S, Amen CR. Host factors in periodontal disease: Periodontal manifestations of Chediak-Higashi syndrome. *J Periodont Res.* 1972; 7:26-35.

53. Cianciola HK, Park BH, Bruck E, Mosovich L, Genco RJ. Prevalence of periodontal disease in insulin-dependent diabetes mellitus (juvenile diabetes). *J Am Dent Assoc.* 1982; 104:653-660.

54. Kisling E, Krebs G. Periodontal conditions in adult patients with mongolism (Down's syndrome). *Acta Odontol Scand.* 1963; 21:391-405.

55. Ingle JI. Paillon-Lefevre syndrome: Precocious periodontosis with associated epidemial lesions. *J Periodontol.* 1959; 30:230-241.

56. Leggott PJ, Robertson PB, Greenspan D, Warea DW, Greenspan JS. Oral manifestations of primary and acquired immunodeficiency diseases in children. *Ped Dent.* 1987; 9:98-104.

57. Page RC, et al. Rapidly progressing periodontitits. A distinct clinical condition. *J Periodontol.* 1983; 54:197-209.

58. Winkler JR, Grassi M, Murray PA. Clinical description and etiology of HIV-associated periodontal diseases. In: Robertson PB, Greenspan JS, eds. *Perspectives on Oral Manifestations of AIDS.* San Diego, Calif. Littleton, Mass.: PSG Publishing Co., Inc. 1988; 49.

59. Winkler JR, Murray PA, Grassi M, Hammerle C. Diagnosis and management of HIV-associated periodontal lesions. *J Amer Dent Assoc.* 1989; Nov Suppl:25-34.

60. Williams CA, Winkler JR, Grassi M, Murray PA. HIV-associated periodontitis complicated by necrotizing stomatitis. *Oral Surg.* 1990; 69:351-355.

61. Löe H, Theilade E, Jensen SB. Experimental gingivitis in man. *J Periodontol.* 1965: 36:177-187.

62. Socransky SS. Relationship of bacteria to the etiology of periodontal disease. *J Dent Res.* 1970, (Suppl 2) 49:203-222.

63. Socransky SS. Microbiology of periodontal disease. Present status and future considerations. *J Periodontol.* 1977; 48:497-504.

64. Page RC, Schroeder H. *Periodontitis in man and other animals. A comparative review.* Basel, Switzerland: S. Karger, 1982.

65. Caton J. Periodontal diagnosis and diagnostic aids. In: Nevins M, Becker W, Kornman K. *Proceedings of the World Workshop in Clinical Periodontics.* American Academy of Periodontology. 1989:I-1.

66. Williams R. Periodontal disease. *N Engl J Med.* 1990; 322:373-382.
67. Listgarten MA. Pathogenesis of periodontitis. *J Clin Periodontol.* 1986; 13:418-430.
68. Greenstein G, Caton J. Periodontal disease activity: A critical assessment. *J Periodontol.* 1990; 61:543-552.
69. Mackenzie, IC, Holm-Pedersen P, Karing T. Age changes in the oral mucous membranes and periodontium. In: Holm-Peterse P, Löe H, eds. *Geriatric Dentistry.* Copenhagen: Munksgaard, 1986; 102.
70. Beck et al. Oral health status: Impact of dental students attitude towards the aged. *The Gerontologist.* 1979; 19:580-585.
71. Cunningham MA, Beck JD, Ettinger RL. Dental students self-assessed competence in treating geriatric patients. *Spec Care Dent.* 1984; 4:113-118.
72. Ettinger RL, Beck JD, McLeran H. Geriatric dentistry: The rationale and strategy for its development and implementation in a dental curriculum. *Geront Geriatric Educ.* 1988; 18:149-164.
73. Resiberg B et al. Longitudinal course of normal aging and progressive dementia of the Alzheimer's type: A prospective study of 106 subjects over a 3.6 year mean interval. *Prog Neuro-psychopharmacol Biol Psychiat.* 1986; 10:571-578.
74. Niessen LC, Jones JA. Zocchi M, Gurian B. Dental care for the patient with Alzheimer's disease. *J Am Dent Assoc.* 1985; 110:207-209.
75. Montelaro S. Alzheimer's disease: A growing concern in geriatric dentistry. *Gen Dent.* 1985; 494-497.
76. Niessen LC, Jones JA. Alzheimer's disease: a guide for dental professionals. *Spec Care Dent.* 1986; 6:6-12.
77. Friedlander AH. Jarvik, LF. The dental management of the patient with dementia. *Oral Surg.* 1987; 64:549-553.
78. Brookfield SD. Structuring programs around learner's needs and abilities. In: *Understanding and facilitating adult learning.* San Francisco: Jossey-Bass, 1986; 233-260.
79. Locker D. Dental health education. In: Lewis DW., coordinator and editor, *Preventive Dental Services.* 2nd ed. 1988 Dept. of National Health and Welfare, Canada.
80. Crall JJ. Information futures in dental education and research: quality assurance. *J Dent Ed.* 1991; 55:257-261.
81. Learman LA et al. Pygmalion in nursing home: the effect of caregive expectations on patient outcomes. *J Am Geriatric Soc.* 1990; 38:797-803.
82. Lund AK, Kegeles SS, Wisenberg M. Motivation techniques for acceptance of preventive health measures. *Med Care.* 1977; 15:678-692, and AK, Kegeles SS, Wisenberg M. Motivation techniques for acceptance of preventive health measures. *Med Care.* 1977; 15:678-6.

Chapter 17
New Research Directions in Gerontological Aspects of Periodontology

Walter J. Loesche, Bruce J. Baum and Marc W. Heft

I. Introduction

The size of the older segment of the population will continue to rise, so that by the year 2030, one-fifth of the U.S. population, i.e., 64 million people, will be 65 years of age. Similar proportions will exist in the populations found in Canada, Western Europe and Japan. The dental health problems of these older individuals will increase in a disproportionate fashion, mainly due to increased retention of teeth and the "polypharmacia" that is used for the medical treatment of many of these individuals. The combination of more teeth and the increased usage of medications that reduce salivary flow suggests that dental caries, including both coronal and root surface decay, will increase. As more teeth are retained and as individuals lose their ability to maintain good oral hygiene, it would seem inevitable that periodontal disease will also increase. However, this does not appear to be the case.

II. The Decline in the Prevalence of Periodontal Disease (M. Heft)

Recent findings have suggested that the prevalence of severe periodontitis in adults is not as great as was believed.[1-6] Further, reports have identified only relatively small subsamples of individuals with disease.[1, 6-11] However, older persons have been found to have a higher prevalence of moderate and severe disease than younger persons.[2,4,7,9,11]

Traditionally, the prevalence of periodontitis has been reported as mean values in subjects or groups of subjects. More recently, investigators have recognized that mean values are inadequate in describing the nature of periodontal disease in populations because of marked intrasubject and intersubject variation.[6,7,9,13] Carlos *et al.*[14] have proposed the Extent and Severity Index (ESI) to describe the extent (mean percent of sites per subject which exceed a threshold level) and severity (mean attachment loss from the CEJ) of periodontal disease in epidemiological surveys.

The well-documented increase in the number of older adults in the U.S., as well as their increased retention of teeth, has made understanding of the epidemiology of oral diseases (including periodontal diseases) in older U.S. and Canadian adults more compelling. In 1985, the National Institute of Dental Research commissioned the National Survey of Oral Health in U.S. Employed Adults and Seniors (NSOH) to characterize the oral health of adults and older adults in the U.S.[4] The latter group was sampled from among those who attend senior centres (defined as "community facilities where older persons come together for services and activities such as educational programs, creative arts, health services or work").

In September, 1985, we initiated a study of elderly Floridians attending senior centres in the six Florida counties which comprise more than half of Florida's 65+ years population (roughly 4% of the U.S. elderly). The study included the same clinical measures as were employed in the NSOH as well as a clinical questionnaire.[1,15] Nine hundred and forty-nine subjects aged 65+ years were examined at 14 sites. Clinical measures (on all teeth excluding third molars) included: coronal and cervical caries (new and recurrent lesions and restorations) and pocketing, attachment loss, calculus, and bleeding measures. The latter periodontal measures were taken from both mesial and buccal sites in two quadrants per subject.

The mean age of the subjects was 76.5 years and 11% were aged 85+ years (older than the NSOH[4]). The mean number of remaining teeth among the 671 dentate individuals was 17.0, and the older individuals had significantly fewer teeth. In the NSOH, 47% of the seniors had ≥ 1 site with bleeding gingiva compared with 66% in the Florida study. Similarly, 10% of the sites probed bled in the NSOH compared with 25% in the Florida study. However, the percent of subjects and mean percent of sites with calculus was greater for NSOH (NSOH: 66% subjects and 54% sites vs. F: 55% subjects and 32% sites).

With regard to gingival recession, the mean recession for the Florida study was 1.4 mm and 62% sites exhibited recession, while in NSOH, the mean recession was 2.1 mm and only 39% of the sites exhibited recession. The mean attachment loss and pocketing was also greater for the Florida group (attachment: F 3.5 mm vs. NSOH 3.2 mm, pocketing: F 2.1 vs. 1.4 mm). Twenty-four percent of the Florida sample had ≥ 1 site with attachment ≥ 7 mm compared with 21% for NSOH.

Sites with severe attachment loss were typically not accompanied by severe pockets in the Florida study, rather with attachment loss, recession apparently increased without a substantial increase in pocket depth. Similar findings have been reported by other investigators.[9,13,17] These findings support the conclusion that many older adults have a history of moderate disease activity, but severe disease is evident in a much smaller segment of the population.

These figures indicate that periodontal disease in the elderly is not as prevalent as initially surmised or that it is on the decline from previous generations. If new research directions are to be explored in periodontal disease, they may have to go beyond or even away from our traditional concepts of periodontal research. In this workshop, we have explored the possibility that good oral and periodontal health is important and, possibly, critical for good medical health in the elderly. In particular, we have discussed salivary gland function in the elderly and led from this into a discussion of how xerostomia may play the key role between periodontal disease and aspiration pneumonia in the elderly. Aspiration pneumonia is a major cause of death in the elderly, so that, if good periodontal health can reduce the prevalence of aspiration pneumonia, this would have an immediate effect on the longevity of the elderly.

III. Salivary Gland Function in the Elderly (B. Baum)

Saliva plays a critical role in maintaining oral health. Salivary components mediate such diverse processes as mucosal lubrication, dental remineralization, antimicrobial action, soft tissue repair, and gustation.[18, 19] In the absence of adequate salivary gland secretion, these functions are compromised, and individuals can suffer multiple morbid consequences.[20]

A common generalization associated with aging is that salivary gland secretion is reduced.[21, 22] This perspective is, however, based on results from early studies which now may be viewed as flawed, primarily because of subject selection. Thus, when residents of nursing homes or clinic patients were used as a source of older subjects, their saliva production levels were greatly reduced when compared with healthy young adults.[23, 24] Relatively recent studies in which salivary secretion has been examined in healthy, non-medicated persons over a wide age range have shown that major salivary gland function is generally well maintained throughout life.[25, 28] Salivary secretion rates (parotid, submandibular; resting, stimulated) are quite variable (10-100-fold range) among healthy persons, and that variability appears to be maintained with increased age.[29]

While no change in saliva production among elders has been observed, it is interesting that several studies have demonstrated that the salivary glands of elderly persons display a marked loss ($\approx$20-40%) in the proportion of acinar cells present.[30-32] Acinar cells are believed to be the only site of fluid secretion in salivary glands.[33, 34] Thus, a paradox is apparent; how do older persons make comparable levels of saliva, when compared to young adults, if their salivary glands contain less functional parenchyma? This has been answered, but not unequivocally proven, by invoking the concept of a reserve secretory capacity,[35] i.e., younger persons contain substantially more acinar tissue than is needed for "normal" salivary secretion. Conceptually, one can view this reserve capacity as being diminished with age and, accordingly, the older person as having a reduced capacity to resist insults to gland parenchyma.

The primary source of such insults would come from iatrogenic effects on gland performance. Thus, many pharmaceuticals (anti-depressants, anti-cholinergics, anti-hypertensives, etc.[36]) or oncologic therapies (e.g., head and neck radiation[37]) can adversely affect salivary flow rates. The conditions which require such therapeutic manoeuvres are much more common among elderly persons than young individuals. Also, a fairly common disease which reduces salivary secretion is the autoimmune exocrinopathy, Sjogren's syndrome. This condition may affect $\approx$1 million post-menopausal persons in the United States.[38] Therefore, it seems likely that the generalization about diminished salivary secretion among the elderly primarily has its application among older persons with systemic disease.[39]

Reduced saliva production in any age group results in comparable symptoms and signs.[20] Xerostomia is the subjective complaint of a dry mouth and is associated with salivary hypofunction, while increased rates of dental caries and difficulty swallowing (especially dry foods) are common objective indicators. Treatment of salivary hypofunction is similar regardless of patient age.[40-42] If there is no parenchymal tissue remaining, which may occur following full irradiation of the salivary glands, then only the use of salivary substitutes and dental prophylactic procedures are presently available. While this approach can greatly reduce dental caries experience,[41] it does little for soft tissue problems.[43] However, if some functional gland parenchyma is present, the reduced secretion can be increased by utilization of a systemically administered secretogogue such as pilocarpine.[40, 44] Use of such a stimulatory agent absolutely requires the presence of some acinar epithelial cells, as other cell types are unable to transport fluid. If use of an autonomic drug is contraindicated, patients with functional gland tissue should still benefit from less-convenient-to-use masticatory and gustatory stimuli (sugarless chewing gum or candy). Finally, if decreased salivary flow rates are related to the use of a prescription medication, then it may be possible to alter the class of drug utilized, change the dosing schedule, or reduce dosage levels.

IV. Aspiration Pneumonia (AP) — (W. Loesche)

Even more ominous for the general health of the individual may be the interaction between periodontal disease and xerostomia, which could predispose the individual to aspiration pneumonia (AP).

The elderly are particularly susceptible to a pneumonia that is secondary to the aspiration of foreign materials, especially oropharyngeal secretions (saliva) and food into the lungs.[45] Among hospitalized elderly patients, pneumonia is associated with a 40% mortality rate.[46] Known risk factors are severe debilitation, recent usage of antibiotics, and the colonization of the oropharyngeal surfaces by aerobic gram-negative bacilli (GNB).[47, 49, 54]

The most intriguing of these risk factors are the GNB. These organisms are not normally inhabitants of the oropharyngeal surfaces, so that their presence on these surfaces is of interest both from the perspective of mucous membrane microbial ecology and as a risk factor for AP. The recent usage of antibiotics could select for these organisms, thereby increasing their levels in any material that is aspirated. But this would not explain why or how these organisms came to be on the oropharyngeal surfaces. Do the GNB come from exogenous sources via the mouth, or do they arrive retrograde from the intestine? The prevailing opinion is that they originate from the intestinal tract, via regurgitation of stomach contents, but evidence for this is almost nonexistent. It is equally possible that the GNB actually originate from exogenous sources such as the diet and that oral environmental conditions that are prevalent in the elderly could lead to the colonization of oral surfaces by these organisms.

The whole saliva of healthy individuals is bereft of detectable GNB, but these organisms are commonly found in older hospitalized individuals.[47, 49] The colonization in the hospitalized individuals has been attributed to the high level of GNB in the hospital environment and to the fact that many of these individuals have recently been treated with antibiotics. However, there could be other factors operating in the hospital environment, such as salivary hypofunction due to the multiple medication regimen that many of these patients are on plus a deplorable lack of oral hygiene.

The salivary hypofunction could predispose these individuals to profound changes in the oral flora. The normal cleansing action of the saliva on the teeth and other oral surfaces is reduced, leading to bacterial accumulations on these surfaces. Also, if the individual exhibits poor oral hygiene, as would be common in the elderly and in the hospitalized, then it is possible in some individuals for the proteolytic organisms, typical of a periodontal disease-associated flora,[50, 51] to become dominant in both the subgingival and supragingival plaque. Several members of this flora, namely *Treponema denticola* and *Porphyromonas gingivalis*, possess a trypsin-like enzyme and also degrade fibronectin.[51] Various investigations have found that the GNB cannot adhere to fibronectin-coated epithelial cell surfaces and, presumably, this coating, under conditions of oral health, prevents the attachment of GNB to the oral epithelial cells in vivo.[52] In fact, there appears to be less fibronectin on the surfaces of buccal epithelial cells obtained from individuals known to be colonized by GNB.

Could it be that the salivary hypofunction predisposes to the overgrowth of a proteolytic (periodontopathic) flora on the teeth and oral surfaces and that this flora, in turn, strips off the "protective" fibronectin coating of the epithelial cells, thereby enabling the GNB to colonize? Indeed, saliva obtained from patients colonized by GNB contained more protease activity than saliva obtained from noncolonised subjects.[53] Treatment of buccal cells from normal subjects *in vitro* with this saliva resulted in decreased cell surface fibronectin and increased adherence of GNB to these cells compared to suitable controls.[52]

These findings support the hypothesis that an increase in the oral proteolytic flora, as measured by salivary protease activity, could be a predisposing factor to the colonization of the oral pharyngeal surfaces by the GNB.

V. The Oral Connection

The known medical risk factors for AP, i.e., being bedridden and being on antibiotics (Figure 1), provide few insights into the prevention of AP. The concern over GNB has lead to the increasing use of potent broad-spectrum antibiotics, such as the extended-spectrum penicillins and cephalosporins, as empirical therapy for many pneumonias,[54] but whether they will have an effect on the incidence of AP remains to be documented. Perhaps, meaningful prevention could be achieved by addressing the conditions prior to debilitation that could have an effect on the colonization of the GNB, namely, the health of the teeth in the ambulatory patient (Figure 1).

A. Teeth vs. No Teeth
It is difficult to obtain suitable specimens for culturing in pneumonia due to the contamination of the sputum with saliva, so that most, if not all, samples are contaminated with the "normal oral flora". Bartlett and Gorbach[55] avoided this contamination by collecting transtracheal aspirates from individuals diagnosed as having aspiration pneumonia. Uniquely oral organisms accounted for 78% of the isolates obtained from 70 patients, whereas GNB accounted for 16% and *Bacteroides fragilis* for 6% of the isolates (Table 1). The four most numerous groups, peptostreptococci, black pigmented bacteroides, *Fusobacterium nucleatum*, and peptococci, are mainly associated with dental plaque and are known to increase in numbers when an individual has periodontal disease.[50, 56] As such, this study suggested that the bacteria resident on the teeth could be the origin of about 65% of the species isolated from pneumonia. If this be the case, then there should be some association between the presence of teeth and aspiration pneumonia.

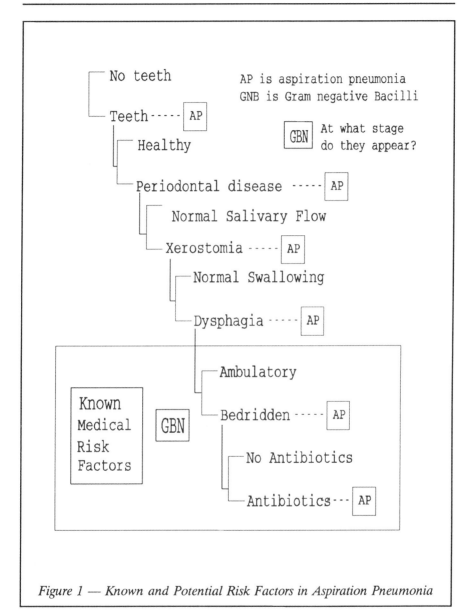

Figure 1 — Known and Potential Risk Factors in Aspiration Pneumonia

Table 1 — Bacteriology of Aspiration Pneumonia

Species	No. of Isolates	Teeth	Periodontal Disease	Oral	G.I.
Anaerobic					
Peptostreptocci	32	+	+ +	+	
Blk. Pigmented Bacteroides	27	+	+ +	+	
F. nucleatum	19	+	+ +	+	
Peptococci	17	+	+ +	+	
B. fragilis	10				+
B. oralis	9	+	+	+	
Facultative					
S. pneumoniae	11			+	
S. aureus	11			+	
Klebsiella	8			(+)	+
Pseudomonas sp.	7			(+)	+
E. coli	6			(+)	+

(+)   Not primary location
Adapted from Bartlett & Gorbach 1974

Evidence for this association has not been sought until the present time, when Limeback found that about 60% of the dentate elderly in the Metro Toronto nursing homes that he surveyed died with a diagnosis of pneumonia, whereas only 40% of the edentulous elderly died of pneumonia (p < 0.05).[57] He also found that there was a significant negative correlation between the total number of dental visits by nursing home residents and the incidence of death due to pneumonia, i.e., the more visits, the fewer numbers of deaths (Limeback, personal communication). His initial findings suggest that the presence of teeth are a liability for the elderly individual because somehow they place him/her at risk for death due to pneumonia.

B. Healthy Teeth vs. Periodontally Diseased Teeth
Why should this be? Teeth should improve the overall quality of life, both due to better masticatory function and to the sense of well-being that comes from the better aesthetics and confidence associated with having one's own teeth. However, the teeth have the only surfaces in the body that do not shed, so that bacterial accumulations on their surfaces can become quite large in the absence of adequate cleansing procedures. Salivary hypofunction could reduce the natural cleaning of the oral cavity, and if this is combined with poor oral hygiene, then considerable numbers of bacteria could accumulate on the tooth surfaces. This scenario occurs each morning when one wakes from sleep after a night of reduced flow of saliva (salivary flow almost ceases during sleep) and no oral hygiene. The numbers of bacteria found in the saliva upon waking are 10 to 20 times that obtained from the same individual during the day.[58]

This increase in bacterial numbers could be even more exaggerated in a xerostomic individual with poor oral hygiene, and could lead to changes in the bacterial composition of the oral flora, such as a selection for GNB, that would have adverse consequences for the health of the individual. Some evidence for a relationship between poor oral hygiene and death due to pneumonia were obtained by Limeback.[57] He devised an Oral Health Status Score that was low if the individuals had no teeth and high if the individuals had a history of dental abscesses. Individuals who died with pneumonia had a significantly higher score than those who died without pneumonia, suggesting that poor oral hygiene could be correlated with the prevalence of pneumonia at death. Is this a gratuitous finding or can it be explained by changes in the oral flora?

Woods and his associates[52, 53] demonstrated that cells of *P. aeruginosa*, one of the more frequently encountered GNB in AP, attached *in vitro* in higher numbers to oral epithelial cells obtained from patients from intensive care units than they did to epithelial cells obtained from healthy volunteers. They studied this phenomenon prospectively in patients undergoing open heart surgery and showed that an increase in the level of salivary proteases post-surgery could be associated with 1) increased adherence of *Ps. aeruginosa* to epithelial cells *in vitro*, and 2) with the actual colonization of *Ps. aeruginosa in vivo*. The source of the proteases was not identified, but it was suggested that they could be derived from inflammatory cells, epithelial cells, or from the normal oral flora.

Of these, the normal oral flora would seem most likely to be the source, as oral hygiene essentially ceases in the intensive care unit, and many of the anaerobic organisms that would be selected for in the stagnant plaque environment would be proteolytic.[51] Also, the xerostomia from the medications and lack of masticatory stimuli could lead to a concentration of this proteolytic activity in the saliva. The magnitude of this increase in proteolytic activity can be deduced from the observation that saliva obtained upon awakening in the morning, and prior to tooth brushing, had significantly more fibronectin-degrading activity/mL saliva than did the saliva collected from the same individuals after toothbrushing.[58] If this were so for normal healthy individuals upon wakening in the morning, one can imagine how much more salivary proteolytic activity would be derived from several days of no oral hygiene in a xerostomic individual, especially if he/she has periodontal disease.

C. Normal Saliva Flow vs. Xerostomia
As noted above, as the volume of saliva decreases, the bacterial density of the residual saliva increases, but this would not, "a priori" lead to fundamental changes in the types of organisms found in the oral flora. However, in both Sjogren's syndrome and in radiation xerostomia, there is a selection for GNB.[59, 60] These chance observations indicate that salivary hypofunction predisposes to the overgrowth of a proteolytic flora on the teeth and oral surfaces and that this flora could, in turn, strip off the "protective" fibronectin coating of the epithelial cells, thereby enabling the GNB to colonize the oral surfaces. These observations support the hypothesis that an increase in the oral proteolytic flora, as measured by salivary protease activity, is a predisposing factor for AP. As such, both the maintenance of dental health and salivary flow would be important prophylactic measures for the prevention of AP. This hypothesis suggests that there could be a connection between periodontal disease, the xerostomia resulting from salivary gland hypofunction, and medical health in the elderly, and if so, this would represent a new research direction in periodontology.

VII. Discussion

There was a question as to the origin of fibronectin and whether it was secreted in the saliva. Fibronectin is secreted in the saliva and formed by the epithelial cells. Any fibronectin found in the gingival crevicular fluid (gcf) would most likely be derived from the serum. This fibronectin would probably have a very short half-life in the gcf, as bacterial enzymes in the plaque would degrade it. A question was raised as to whether pilocarpine would be available in a slow-release device. The answer was a tentative no because it is unlikely that a commercial sponsor could obtain patent protection. Also, as pilocarpine is so inexpensive and convenient to take orally, there seems to be no need for a slow-release devise. It was noted that the salivary substitutes on the market provide good protection against enamel demineralization but that there was a need for a salivary substitute that provided adequate lubrication for xerostomic patients.

There were several questions and comments in both the workshop and plenary session related to the possible connection between poor oral hygiene, periodontal disease and aspiration pneumonia. One individual expressed the opinion that, if there was, indeed, such a relationship, it should be addressed quickly, lest apathy set in. There was some discussion as to whether good dental health was an issue, which hospital and nursing home administrators wanted to address. It was stated that these individuals would not look favourably towards any treatments that would unnecessarily increase their operating expenses. Thus, it will be necessary to obtain adequate scientific data which shows that good oral health predisposes to good medical health.

Some individuals expressed disappointment that other areas of periodontal research were not addressed. Among these were the role of the immune system in periodontal disease. It is well known that the competence of the immune system declines with aging. The question was raised as to whether the retention of teeth—especially, teeth with large plaque accumulates—are an even greater challenge to a diminished immune system. One individual wondered how the inflammatory processes would be affected in the older individual with teeth and poor oral hygiene. Would inflammatory mediators such as the prostaglandins behave in the same way or would there be an altered metabolism related to aging. One individual expressed disappointment that research into new and better health care delivery systems were not described.

Acknowledgements

Dr. Loesche's research for this paper was supported by U.S.P.H.S. grant no. DE09142 from the National Institute of Dental Research.

Endnotes

1.   Gilbert GH, Heft MW. Periodontal status of older Floridians attending senior activity centres. *J. Clin. Periodontol.* in press (Issue 4, 1992).

2.   Hunt RJ, Field HM, Beck JD. The prevalence of periodontal conditions in a non-institutionalized elderly population. *Gerodontics* 1: 176-180, 1985.

3.   Ismail AI, Eklund SA, Striffler DF, Szpunar SM. The prevalence of advanced loss of periodontal attachment in two New Mexico populations. *J. Periodont. Res.* 22: 119-124, 1986.

4.   Miller AJ, Brunelle JA, Carlos JP, Brown LJ, Löe H. Oral health of U.S. adults. The national survey of oral health in U.S. employed adults and seniors: 1985-1986. Washington, D.C.: *National Institute of Dental Research,* 1987; Publication no. (NIH) 87-2868.

5.   Capilouto ML, Douglas CW. Trends in the prevalence and severity of periodontal diseases in the U.S: a public health problem? *J. Publ. Health Dent.* 48: 245-251, 1988.

6.   Johnson NW, Griffiths GS, Wilton JMA, Maiden MFJ, Curtis MA, Gillett IR, Wilson DT, Sterne JAC. Detection of high-risk groups and individuals for periodontal diseases: evidence for the existence of high-risk groups and individuals and approaches to their detection. *J. Clin. Periodontol.* 15: 276-282, 1988.

7.   Hugoson A, Jordan T. Frequency distribution of individuals aged 20-70 years according to severity of periodontal disease. *Community Dentistry and Oral Epidemiol.* 10: 187-192, 1982.

8.   Beck JD, Lainson PA, Field HM, Hawkins, BF. Risk factors for various levels of periodontal disease and treatment needs in Iowa. *Community Dentistry and Oral Epidemiol.* 12: 17-22, 1984.

9.   Löe H, Anerud A, Boysen H, Morrison E. Natural history of periodontal disease in man. Rapid, moderate, and no loss of attachment in Sri Lankan Laborers to 46 years of age. *J. Clin. Periodontol.* 13: 431-440, 1986.

10.   Okamoto H, Yoneyama T, Lindhe J, Haffajee A, Socransky S. Methods of evaluating periodontal disease data in epidemiological research. *J. Clin. Periodontol.* 15: 430-439, 1988.

11.   Schurch E Jr., Minder CE, Lang NP, Geering AH. Periodontal conditions in a randomly selected population in Switzerland. *Community Dentistry and Oral Epidemiol.* 16: 181-186, 1988.

12.   Ismail AI, Morrison EC, Burt BA, Caffesse RG, Kavanagh MT. Natural history of periodontal disease in adults: findings from the Tecumseh periodontal disease study, 1959-1987. *J. Dent. Res.* 69: 430-435, 1990.

13.   Yoneyama T, Okamoto H, Lindhe J, Socransky SS, Haffajee AD. Probing depth, attachment loss and gingival recession: findings from a clinical examination in Ushiku, Japan. *J. Clin. Periodontol.* 15: 581-591, 1988.

14.   Carlos JP, Wolfe MD, Kingman A. The extent and severity index: a simple method for use in epidemilogical studies of periodontal disease. *J. Clin. Periodontol.* 13: 500-505, 1986.

15.   Heft MW, Gilbert GH. Tooth loss and caries prevalence in older Floridians attending senior activity centers. *Community Dentistry and Oral Epidemiol.* in press.

16.   Goodson JM. Selection of suitable indicators of periodontitis. In: Bader, J. ed. *Risk assessment in dentistry.* Chapel Hill, N.C: UNC Dental Ecology, 69-74, 1990.

17.   Gunsolley JC, Best AM. Change in attachment level. *J. Periodontol.* 59: 450-456, 1988.

18.   Mandel ID. The function of saliva. *J. Dent. Res.* 66: 623-627, 1987.

19.   Mandel ID. The role of saliva in maintaining oral homeostasis. *JADA* 119: 298-304, 1989.

20.   Fox PC, Van der Ven PF, Sonies BC, Weiffenbach JM, Baum BJ. Xerostomia: evaluation of a symptom with increasing significance. *JADA* 110: 519-529, 1985.

21.   Baum BJ. Research on aging and oral health: an assessment of current status and future needs. *Spec. Care Dent.* 1: 156-165, 1981

22.   Baum BJ. Salivary gland fluid secretion during aging. *J. Amer. Geriatics Soc.* 37: 453-458, 1989.

23.   Meyer J, Necheles H. Studies in old age. IV. The clinical significance of salivary, gastric and pancreatic secretion in the aged. *JAMA* 115: 2050-2053, 1940.

24.   Bertram U. Xerostomia. *Acta Odont. Scand.* 25 (Suppl 49): 1-126, 1967.

25.   Baum BJ. Evaluation of stimulated parotid saliva flow rate in different age groups. *J. Dent. Res.* 60: 1292-1296, 1981.

26.   Chauncey HH, Borkan G, Wayler A, Feller RP, Kapur KK. Parotid fluid composition in healthy males. *Adv. Physiol. Sci.* 28: 323-328, 1981.

27.   Tylenda CA, Ship JA, Fox PC, Baum BJ. Evaluation of submandibular salivary flow rate in different age groups. *J. Dent. Res.* 67: 1225-1228, 1988.

28.   Ship JA, Baum BJ. Is salivary flow reduced in old people? *Lancet* 336: 1507, 1990.

29.   Ship JA, Fox PC, Baum BJ. How much saliva is enough? *JADA* 122: 63-69, 1991.

30. Waterhouse JP, Chisholm DM, Winter RB, Patel M, Yale RS. Replacement of functional parenchymal cells by fat and connective tissue in human submandibular salivary glands. *J. Oral Pathol.* 2: 16-27, 1973.
31. Scott J. Quantitative age changes in the histological structure of human submandibular salivary glands. *Arch. Oral Biol.* 22: 221-227, 1977.
32. Scott J, Flower EA, Burns J. A quantitative study of histological changes in the human parotid gland occurring with adult age. *J. Oral Pathol.* 16: 505-510, 1987.
33. Young JA, Van Lennep EW. Salivary and salt glands. In: Giebisch G. Tosteson DC, Ussing HH (eds) *Membrane Transport in Biology*, Berlin, Springer Verlag, 1979, pp. 563-674.
34. Baum BJ. Neurotransmitter control of secretion. *J. Dent. Res.* 66: 628-632, 1987.
35. Scott J. Structural changes in salivary glands. In: Ferguson DB (ed) *The Aging Mouth*, Basel, Karger, 1987, pp. 40-62.
36. Sreebny LM, Schwartz SS. A reference guide to drugs and dry mouth. *Gerodontology* 5: 75-99, 1986.
37. Anderson MW, Izutsu KT, Rice JC. Parotid gland pathophysiology following mixed gamma and neutron irradiation of cancer patients. *Oral Surg.* 52: 495-500, 1981.
38. Talal N. Overview of Sjogren's syndrome. *J. Dent. Res.* 66: 672-674, 1987.
39. Baum BJ. Dental and oral disorders. In: Abrams WB, Fletcher AJ (eds) *The Merck Manual of Geriatrics*, Rahway, NJ, Merck & Co., pp. 466-475, 1990.
40. Fox PC. Systemic therapy for salivary gland hypofunction. *J. Dent. Res.* 66: 689-692, 1987.
41. Wright WE. Management of oral sequelae. *J. Dent. Res.* 66: 699-702, 1987.
42. Sreebny LM. Salivary flow in health and disease. *Compend. Cont. Educ. Dent. Suppl.* 13: S461-S469, 1989.
43. Hatton MN, Levine MJ, Margarone JE, Aguirre A. Lubrication and viscosity features of human saliva and commercially available saliva substitutes. *J. Oral Maxillofac. Surg.* 45: 496-499, 1987.
44. Fox PC, Van der Ven PF, Baum BJ, Mandel ID. Pilocarpine for the treatment of xerostomia associated with salivary gland dysfunction. *Oral Surg.* 61: 243-245, 1986.
45. Schneider EL. Infectious diseases in the elderly. *Ann. Intern. Med.* 98:395-400, 1983.
46. Fang G-D, Fine M, Orloff J, Arisumi D, Yu VL, Kapoor W, Grayston JT, Wang SP, Kohler R, Muder RR, Yee YC, Rihs JD, Vickers RM. New and emerging etiologies for community-acquired pneumonia with implications for therapy. *Med.* 69:307-316, 1990.

47. Johanson WG Jr., Pierce AK, Sanford JP. Changing pharyngeal bacterial flora of hospitalized patients: emergence of gram- negative bacilli. *N. Eng. J. Med.* 281: 1969.

48. Gonzalez CL, Calia FM. Bacteriologic flora of aspiration induced pulmonary infections. *Arch. of Intern. Med.* 135: 711-714, 1975.

49. LaForce FM. Hospital-acquired gram-negative rod pneumonias. *Amer. J. Med.* 70:664-669, 1981.

50. Loesche WJ, Syed SA, Schmidt E, Morrison EC. Bacterial profiles of subgingival plaques in periodontitis. *J. Periodontol.* 56:447-456, 1985.

51. Wikstrom M, Linde A. Ability of oral bacteria to degrade fibronectin. *Infect Immun.* 51:707-711, 1986.

52. Woods DE, Straus DC, Johanson WG Jr., Bass JA. Role of fibronectin in the prevention of adherence of Pseudomonas aeruginosa to buccal cells. *J. Inf. Dis.* 143:784-790, 1981.

53. Woods DE, Straus DC, Johanson WG Jr., Bass JA. Role of salivary protease activity in adherence to gram-negative bacilli to mammalian buccal epithelial cells in vivo. *J. Clin. Invest.* 68:1435-1440, 1981.

54. Grasela TH, Timm E, Welage L. A nationwide survey of antibiotic utilization of antibiotic utilization in bacterial pneumonia (abstract). *Intersci Conf Antimicrob Ag Chemother.* 28:761, 1988.

55. Bartlett JG, Gorbach SL, Finegold SM. The bacteriology of aspiration pneumonia. *Amer. J. Med.* 56:202-207, 1974.

56. Moore WEC. Microbiology of periodontal disease. *J. Periodontol. Res.* 22:335-341, 1987.

57. Limeback H. The relationship between oral health and systemic infections among elderly residents of chronic care facilities: A review. *Gerondont.* 7: 131-137, 1988.

58. Gibbons RJ, Etherden I. Fibronectin-degrading enzymes in saliva and their relationship to oral cleanliness. *J. Periodont. Res.* 21: 386-395, 1986.

59. Brown LR, Dreizen S, Handler S. Effects of selected caries preventive regimens on microbial changes following irradiation induced xerostomia in cancer patients. *Proc. Microbiological Aspects of Dental Caries. Sp. Suppl. Microbiol. Abst.* 1:275-290, 1976.

60. Ayars GH, Altman LC, Fretwell MD. Effect of decreased salivation and pH on the adherence of Klebsiella species to human buccal epithelial cells. *Infect. Immun.* 38:179-182, 1982.

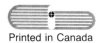
Printed in Canada